Choleste
high blood cholester~ .... cause of coronary
heart disease leading to heart attacks. It is established
beyond doubt that lowering elevated cholesterol
level decreases the risk of heart attacks. Studies
show that every 1% reduction in cholesterol level
leads to 2% reduction in the risk of heart disease.

The theme of this book is preventing coronary heart
disease by recognizing, modifying and reducing the
risk due to high blood cholesterol. While many of us
are aware of the risk, few really know whether they
are in the high, medium or low risk category. This
book takes away your fears but cautions you; it
reveals the likely damages caused by high
cholesterol, and shows you the way to counter them.
It tells you how simple changes in diet and lifestyle
can bring cholesterol within normal limits.

Informative, authoritative and comprehensive —
High Blood Cholesterol is backed by the latest in
research findings, surgical remedies and medicinal
cures.

The Author

Dr. Krishan Gupta is Professor of Medicine at the New York Medical College and a fellow of the Royal College of Physicians (UK), American College of Physician, New York Academy of Medicine and the Gerontological Society of America. A National and University Merit List Scholarship holder, Dr. Gupta completed his MBBS from Punjab University, and has held prestigious appointments in the UK, including that of consultant physician in England.

Dr. Gupta is an acknowledged authority in Internal Medicine and Geriatrics. His conviction that people should possess a working knowledge and an intelligent understanding of modern day diseases has been the motivating factor behind his authorship of numerous books, medical articles and book chapters. Although he is concerned with the recovery of health, he places equal importance on the prevention of disease. The question-answer style that he frequently adopts provides the reader with answer to doubts or questions often left unanswered by doctors.

High Blood Cholesterol

Causes, Prevention and Treatment

Dr Krishan Gupta
MD, FRCP, FACP
Professor of Medicine
New York Medical College, USA

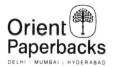

Orient
Paperbacks
DELHI | MUMBAI | HYDERABAD

In memory of
My Father and Uncle

www.orientpaperbacks.com

ISBN : 978-81-222-0166-6

1st Published 1996
9th Printing 2011

High Blood Cholesterol: Causes, Prevention & Treatment

© Krishan Gupta

Cover design by Vision Studio

Published by
Orient Paperbacks
(A division of Vision Books Pvt. Ltd.)
5A/8, Ansari Road, New Delhi-110 002

Printed in India at
Saurabh Printers Pvt. Ltd., Noida

Cover Printed at
Ravindra Printing Press, Delhi-110 006

Foreword

Heart disease remains the leading cause of death and lost productivity in most parts of the world. In the United States alone, over 50 billion US dollars are spent each year treating heart disease and its complications with millions of persons unnecessarily suffering from pain, days away from work, and diminished quality of life. Diet, exercise and lifestyle have all been shown capable of influencing one's individual genetic predisposition to developing heart disease. Although we now appreciate that no one factor is responsible for the alteration that results in 'blocked' blood vessels, the role of cholesterol and its potential danger is one that cannot be forgotten. In fact, the more we know about our cholesterol and ways of keeping it under control, the better will we be able to escape from heart disease. What many people are not aware of, however, is the serious effect that high cholesterol may have on other body functions. A direct link has been demonstrated between cholesterol and one's risk of having a stroke, peripheral vascular disease leading to problems with walking and circulation, reduced kidney function, and blood pressure.

High Blood Cholesterol — Causes, Prevention & Treatment is a must for reading by anyone who wishes to remain healthy. It not only offers a wealth of factual information for the reader, but provides practical information, dietary guidance, and useful tables to refer to. Regardless of your background or level of knowledge regarding cholesterol, this book offers something for you. Only by understanding cholesterol and its potential for causing harm, can we prevent problems from occurring; only by preventing problems, can we eliminate the need for treatment. While you must take the first step, this book provides the path you should follow.

Steven R. Gambert, MD, FACP
*Professor of Medicine and Gerontology,
Associate Dean for Academic Programs,
New York Medical College,
Valhalla, New York.*

Contents

Acknowledgements

I am particularly thankful to my daughter, Shalini, for her valuable suggestions and for tolerating my repeated modifications and updating of the text. Veena, my wife, and Sheila, my other daughter, have been equally helpful in giving their time and support during this project. Special appreciation is due to Mr Sudhir Malhotra (Orient Paperbacks) for his patience, understanding and continuing enthusiasm.

PART I
Understanding Cholesterol

1

Introduction

He who has health, has hope; and he who has hope, has everything.

ARABIAN PROVERB

Coronary heart disease (CHD) continues to be the leading cause of death in many countries. Despite significant success in reducing the death rate by 40% during the past 30 years, approximately 1.5 million adults continue to suffer from a heart attack each year in the United States alone; over half a million of them die each year. The situation is even worse in countries like Canada, England, Germany, France, Holland, Yugoslavia and Russia. There are more heart attacks per 1000 adult population in almost all of these countries as compared to the United States.

The incidence of CHD in India is fast catching up with that of developed countries. Over 24 million suffer from heart ailments in India now. At least 20 million others have diagnosed hypertension or increased blood pressure — a major risk factor for CHD.

Dr P.A. Kale, honorary professor of cardiology, G.S. Medical College and K.E.M. Hospital, Bombay, ranks CHD, as a cause of death, in fourth place behind tuberculosis,

---

1. *Business India* (Aug. 30-Sept. 12, 1993): 122.

communicable diseases and malnutrition. A 1993 survey of the urban Delhi population shows the prevalence of CHD to be 31.9 per thousand adults.

There is concern over the increasing incidence of CHD among people below 40 years in India as compared to people below 50 years in the West. Dr A.B. Mehta, chief of cardiology, Sion Hospital, and consultant cardiologist, Jaslok and Breach Candy Hospitals, says: 'One in ten heart attacks occur in people below 40 years. My youngest patient is 21, with five vessel blockages.'[2]

Dr Natoobhai Shah, senior consultant and cardiologist, Bombay Hospital, presented one of the first studies on younger populations (40 years and below) at the Asian Pacific Congress in Singapore. 'I have found the incidence of CHD in young Indians very much on the rise. From the admission figures at Bombay Hospital, one out of three were 40 years or below — a very alarming ratio, compared to the incidence in the West.[3]

Coronary heart disease is a preventable condition. We do not have to accept heart attacks as an inevitable part of life. How have the Americans succeeded in reducing the death rate due to heart disease over the past 30 years? The answer lies in consistent efforts to educate people to control the risk factors leading to coronary heart disease. Many other developed countries have also launched health education programmes.

I have been particularly interested in observing the thoughts and attitudes of patients from various countries. In fact, it all started with my stay in England from 1973 to 1985. It is typical to see patients from over a dozen different countries if one is running an outpatient clinic in any major hospital in London. What fascinated me most during those years was a wide variation in the patients' thoughts and reactions, the degree of seriousness or sense of neglect towards the issues of health and disease. The thousands of Indian

2 & 3. *Business India* (Aug. 30-Sept. 12, 1993): 122.

patients I interacted with can be broadly placed in three different categories, each reacting somewhat differently to the threat of heart attack and the question of risk factors. Let me share some typical responses with you:

> I have heard of these risk factors and other statistical data regarding diseases, but I am really fine. I don't think that they are in any way related to my life.

> Yes, I believe in these facts—the risk factors are perhaps real but I am used to my own lifestyle. I have managed fairly well so far. Perhaps it is too late at the age of 46. In any case, I have so many other things to take care of. I don't have much time to get into these things. I am just too busy!

> I know people who just eat everything and are still alive at the age of 58 or 62. If they can make it, why can't I?

I am sure you have come across people from each group. They somehow keep postponing their plans to change things. Unfortunately, the same people, when affected by a sudden heart attack, feel so helpless; many blame themselves for the rest of their lives and even become severely depressed. It is, indeed, very important to clearly understand the information and salient scientific facts regarding heart disease and its relationship with high cholesterol. Once you have the facts, it is for you to take a decision and the resultant appropriate action. There is a lot that you can do to reduce your risk of heart attack. Fortunately it is not very difficult. All you need is an interest and willingness to act now!

The purpose of this book is to draw your attention to the serious problem of high cholesterol that makes millions of Indians more prone to heart attacks. Frequent references have been made to recent scientific studies and their conclusions. Everything in this book is based on the findings of numerous scientific studies conducted in many different countries. With the continuing success in the reduction of death rate due to heart disease in the United States and other developed countries, it is only natural to refer to their accomplishments and continuing campaigns against cholesterol.

This book is all about an easy and practical approach to the problem of high cholesterol. Particular attention has been given to the causes of high cholesterol, and how simple changes in your diet, exercise and lifestyle can bring your cholesterol within normal limits. Fortunately, only a small percentage of people with high cholesterol require drug treatment; yet, drugs may be necessary and, indeed, life saving for those who cannot lower their cholesterol levels despite dietary and lifestyle changes. The good news is that even if you have neglected your coronary arteries for all these years, lower cholesterol levels can reverse the damage caused by the fat and cholesterol deposition in your arteries. But it is only from your own awareness and efforts that you can bring down your cholesterol level.

I hope that this book will provide you with practical up-to-date information regarding the threat of high cholesterol and practical methods of reducing it. My primary goal has been to reach the average reader who does not have much of a medical background. Some of the essential terms are explained in the glossary section at the end of the book. Winning the war against cholesterol requires your urgent attention. Good Luck!

2

The Cholesterol Story

The groundwork of all happiness is health.

LEIGH HUNT

The major risk factors for coronary heart disease include smoking, lack of exercise, high blood pressure or hypertension and high blood cholesterol. Smoking has been recognized as a risk factor since the 1950s. The fact that blood pressure reduction was necessary to cut down the risk of heart disease and a stroke has become the focus of attention since 1970.

The cholesterol story is a comparatively recent one. Although scientists and physicians have suspected high cholesterol to be a risk factor for over forty years, it is only during the past decade or so that the results of several scientific studies have already demonstrated a strong relationship between high cholesterol level and heart disease. Furthermore, it has been established that by reducing your cholesterol by 1%, you can reduce your risk of heart disease by upto 2%. A still more remarkable discovery is that you can even reverse the hardening and narrowing of your coronary arteries (atherosclerosis) through a low fat and low cholesterol diet and other changes in your lifestyle.

The National Institute of Health in the United States, for

example, found that people with blood cholesterol readings of over 265 mg were, at least, four times more at risk of CHD as compared to those with readings of 190 mg or less. It has been noted that only a very small percentage of people with cholesterol levels below 160 mg have heart attacks. Large population studies have found a definite and substantial increase in the rate of heart attack in those with blood cholesterol readings of 240 mg and over. Your chances of heart attack start rising significantly if your cholesterol rises over 200 mg[1]. High cholesterol, like high blood pressure, has been termed as a *Silent Killer*, since there are no symptoms of high cholesterol itself.

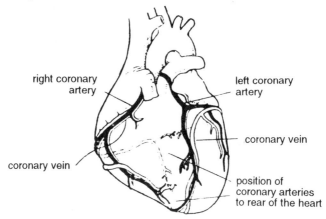

Coronary arteries which supply blood to the heart.

One day, it is possible that your heart may experience lack of oxygen due to insufficient blood supply caused by the slow clogging and blockage of the coronary arteries. This is known as atherosclerosis and is due to the deposition of fat and cholesterol in the walls of your arteries — small-sized pipes that carry blood to different parts of your body, including the heart. If a major artery leading to the heart is completely blocked, this will immediately cut off the blood supply to a

---

1. Desirable cholesterol levels are explained in Chapter 4.

part of the heart and cause a heart attack.

Cholesterol: Changing Attitudes

The following are some of the major studies on cholesterol; the results clearly demonstrate a link between high cholesterol and heart disease:

The Framingham Heart Study, 1952: More than 5,000 adult men and women from Framingham were studied over a period of 30 years. This was the first major study to show that people with lower cholesterol levels were less likely to have heart attacks.

Coronary Drug Project, 1974: More than 8,000 middle-aged men were studied. The conclusion was that a simple medication like nicotinic acid could successfully lower the cholesterol and cut down the chances of death due to heart attacks.

Multiple Risk Factor Intervention Trial (MRFIT), *1982:* More than 12,000 men were studied over a period of 6 years. The conclusion was that if the cholesterol was reduced significantly, the incidence of death rate due to heart disease would be substantially lower.

Lipid Research Clinic's Coronary Primary Prevention Trial, 1984: More than 3,800 middle-aged men with high cholesterol were treated with diet and drugs to reduce cholesterol. The conclusion was that through cholesterol reduction, heart attacks could be reduced by as much as 20%.

Helsinki Heart Study, 1987: More than 4,000 middle-aged men were studied for 5 years. Medication used helped in reducing the cholesterol level and heart attacks.

Cholesterol-lowering Atherosclerosis Study, 1987: In this case, 162 men who had already have heart attacks and bypass operations were studied for a period of 2 years. With diet control and medication use, the narrowing and clogging of the coronary arteries were noted to have been relieved significantly.

These findings highlighted the strong relationship between

19

heart attack and cholesterol, and led the US Department of Health to launch a full-scale war against cholesterol In the United States, the National Cholesterol Education Programme (NCEP) was organized, following the convincing results of several cholesterol studies in the early 1980s.

In my own medical experience, I have seen a great change in our attitudes towards cholesterol. Blood cholesterol results of 250-300 mg were commonly dismissed as normal even in patients with proven heart attacks some twenty years ago. During my 12-year medical practice in England, I must have treated many thousands of patients with hypertension, CHD and other heart problems. Cholesterol checks were routinely done as a part of the blood work in most of these patients. The laboratories commonly reported results up to 300 mg as 'within normal limits'. Even if the results were between 300-400 mg, there was only a mild reaction by the medical community. Few considered it a significantly serious problem. Only those with levels over 400 mg qualified for serious discussion with the physician. Such was the case until the mid and late 1970s.

The awareness in the medical community about the significance of high blood cholesterol, in fact, started with the result of several large population studies carried out in the early 1980s. The National Cholesterol Education Programme was launched by the US Government in the mid 1980s. The American public today regards the threat of high cholesterol as one of their major concerns. Pressure groups and increasing public awareness has recently forced fast food chains like McDonalds and Burger King in the United States to change the fat and cholesterol content of their food items. The awareness of the American public in the area of cholesterol has, perhaps, no match anywhere else in the world. With the experience of treating thousands of patients on both sides of the Atlantic, specifically in the UK and the US, I have often tried to compare notes and ask questions about fat and cholesterol from patients in both countries. Surely the cholesterol awareness of an average American is far more superior.

The US Food and Drug Administration Department requires that most food items in tins and packets must carry information regarding their nutritional contents. It is a common sight to watch people in the big supermarkets looking very carefully at these labels. It is only through these steps that the population there has succeeded in lowering the risk of heart disease.

We, in India, have lagged behind in our efforts. There are many possible reasons for our slowness. Lack of education and resources is a major factor. Our own scientists and physicians have, however, attributed the problem of increasing deaths to CHD and high cholesterol. That, of course, is not enough. There is a paramount need to understand the problem of high cholesterol and to do all that is necessary to control high levels of it. We cannot really afford to be complacent.

Take Charge of Your Health

It is now well established that a persistently high cholesterol level can almost certainly precipitate a catastrophic event such as a heart attack in your life. So the need to take appropriate action is an urgent one. High cholesterol is dangerous for your heart and doing nothing about it may prove to be lethal. You cannot really wait for the government or your own doctor to talk to you about this problem. I admit that physicians all over the world have an obligation to educate their patients regarding important risk factors like high cholesterol but then, don't leave it all to the doctors! Frankly speaking, you have to be in charge of your own health. If you continue to ignore these important matters, you may not even be alive to complain against the government or even a physician. The ultimate responsibility is yours!

During the past twenty years, many people in India have acquired considerable wealth; millions have joined the rapidly expanding middle class. With this growth and prosperity, their lifestyle has, inevitably, become more hectic. Unfortunately, for most people in India, this economic success has failed to generate sufficient interest in health-promoting activities. Most people still do not have an idea of calorific requirements and a balanced diet. Among the affluent groups, obesity is a common problem. In the West, over 50% of all adults take some form of regular exercise, whereas less than 5% of Indians do so. The concept of health clubs is a fairly new one and heard of only in metropolitan cities; so while people in countries like the United States have stopped smoking in large numbers, statistics project an increasing population of smokers in India. With a sedentary lifestyle, inappropriate food habits, smoking, high stress level and, of course, the problem of high cholesterol level, is it really surprising that an increasing number of people are being affected by heart disease!

If you are seriously interested in preventing a heart attack, knowing your exact cholesterol level is the first and foremost step that you must take. Based on your cholesterol results alone, you can place yourself in the high, medium or low risk category for a future heart attack. The next step would be to follow a cholesterol-reducing programme, which alone, can significantly lower your risk of heart attack.

3

What is Cholesterol?

In science we must be interested in things, not in persons.

MARIE CURIE

Cholesterol is a waxy material that is found in many food items including milk, cheese, eggs, butter, *ghee*, fish, beef, pork, chicken and goat meat. It is a naturally occurring, fat-like substance with a complex chemical formula, and is used to build cells and make hormones. Some amount of cholesterol is necessary for the proper functioning of body cells. For example, the presence of cholesterol is essential for the formation of sex hormones and vitamin D metabolism in the body. In young children, cholesterol is required for the development of brain cells. The membranes of many cells require a minimum quantity of cholesterol for healthy functioning.

Sources and Metabolism of Cholesterol

Cholesterol in the blood comes from two main sources:

1. The cholesterol ingested from outside, that is, taken in the daily diet. An average vegetarian consumes between 200-400 mg of cholesterol daily, while a non-vegetarian usually consumes between 400-600 mg of cholesterol.

2. A large part of the cholesterol in the blood comes

from the cholesterol production within the liver; it has been seen that if the oral intake of cholesterol through food is reduced, the liver tends to produce a little extra cholesterol, at least, during the initial few weeks.

The mechanism of metabolism of cholesterol is rather complex and involves several complicated pathways, receptors (sites on the cells that receive a particular substance), and enzyme actions.

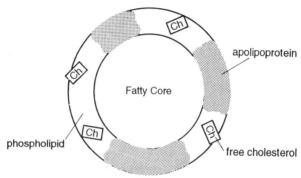

Cross-section of a typical lipoprotein.

Let us look at the way the body handles cholesterol that is ingested through different food items. Cholesterol itself cannot be dissolved in the blood or water. Like many other food particles, after absorption from the intestine, the dietary fat and cholesterol are transferred to the liver for further metabolic action. In the liver, cholesterol combines with water-soluble substances called apolipoproteins and phospholipids to form chylomicrons. Chylomicrons are a form of complex particles called lipoproteins, that is, fats combined with proteins.

Types of Lipoproteins

Three types of lipoproteins carry cholesterol from the liver through the blood circulation to different parts of the body. These three lipoproteins play a major role in causing heart disease. They are distinguished from one another when the blood is centrifuged. Very dense particles settle down and the low density ones remain on top.

Very Low Density Lipoprotein (VLDL): Large fat particles also called chylomicrons, triglycerides and fatty acids form VLDL. As the name suggests, these particles have very low density and weight. Some of the VLDL is used for energy; the other is stored in the fat deposits. A good portion of VLDL is returned to the liver for excretion. VLDL is converted into intermediate density lipoprotein (IDL) and low density lipoprotein (LDL).

Low Density Lipoprotein (LDL): LDL is a product of VLDL, after the removal of the triglycerides. LDL is the most cholesterol-rich lipoprotein in the blood. A portion of LDL is used for fat storage; the rest is sent back to the liver for excretion. Excessive accumulation of LDL in the blood is definitely harmful, since it gets deposited in the walls of the arteries and slowly results in the clogging and narrowing of the arteries. LDL is often referred to as the 'bad' cholesterol. In healthy adults, LDL concentration of over 130 mg/100 ml of blood is considered to be unsafe. The higher the LDL level, the more the danger of a heart attack.

High Density Lipoprotein (HDL): HDL is often referred to as 'good' cholesterol. It is formed in the liver and walls of the small intestine. While maturing in the blood stream, it obtains cholesterol from the surrounding tissues. The blood circulation then transports the HDL back to the liver, from where the cholesterol is excreted in the bile. This is how the HDL cleanses the body and helps a person get rid of excessive amounts of cholesterol. Women, in general, tend to have a higher amount of HDL; that is one of the reasons why women tend to have a lower incidence of heart attack, at least, until the age of menopause. Adults with a HDL level below 35 mg are at a greater risk of heart attack. Those with a HDL level of less than 25 mg may get a serious heart attack even though their total cholesterol level may be within normal limits, that is, less than 200 mg.

Our understanding of the cholesterol metabolism in the body is still in its infancy. Several new types of receptors on the cells and fragments of lipoproteins are currently being looked into by researchers. In 1985, Goldstein and Brown were awarded the Nobel prize for their wonderful discovery of the receptors involved in cholesterol metabolism. It is estimated that between 25-30% of the total population may have some degree of defect in these receptors. The difference in the receptor activity may explain the reason why only some members of the same family consuming a similar diet may have high cholesterol levels, while others do not.

The interrelationship between genetic factors and lipoprotein receptors on the cells is also a comparatively new field of research. It is expected that during the next ten years, our knowledge of cholesterol metabolism will improve significantly. However, while we wait for these new discoveries, we cannot afford to ignore the reality that has already been established—high cholesterol is a killer!

Triglycerides

Triglycerides are a type of fat produced by the liver. They comprise three fatty acids, each attached to a backbone provided

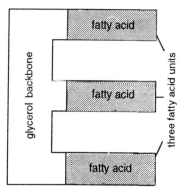

Basic structure of a triglyceride.

by glycerol. Although the high cholesterol and LDL levels have been firmly accepted as the cause of the clogging of the arteries, physicians are less certain about the role of triglycerides. However, results from the famous Framingham Study have recently concluded that high triglyceride level is, in itself, a significant risk factor for coronary heart disease. People who are diabetic, overweight, or have kidney disease are especially seen to have

26

high triglyceride levels. In a normal adult, the triglyceride level is usually between 100-200 mg. If all other results are satisfactory, a mildly-elevated level of triglyceride of up to 300 mg alone, is still not considered very threatening to your arteries. However, readings over 300 mg require treatment with diet, medication or both. In most cases triglycerides are noted to be high only in the presence of other abnormal significant risk

4

Desirable Cholesterol Levels

A single fact is worth a shipload of argument.

PROVERB

Total cholesterol is the sum total of cholesterol carried by three kinds of lipoproteins: very low density lipoprotein (VLDL), low density lipoprotein (LDL) and high density lipoprotein (HDL).

Normal and High Blood Cholesterol Levels

The American categorisations of normal and high total cholesterol levels are, by far, the most comprehensive and widely accepted. The National Cholesterol Education Programme (NCEP) categorised cholesterol levels for adults as given below:

Total Blood Cholesterol Levels

< 200 mg	-	Desirable total blood cholesterol
200-239 mg	-	Borderline high total blood cholesterol
> 240 mg	-	High total blood cholesterol

In recent years, health care agencies in different countries have issued their own recommendations regarding evaluation of normal and high total blood cholesterol levels in adults.

28

These recommendations are, however, more or less the same in different countries.

Besides measuring the total cholesterol, there are three other results relating to HDL, LDL and triglycerides that are of importance for further blood testing for fats.

HDL—The 'Good' Cholesterol: HDL is often referred to as 'good cholesterol' and LDL is commonly referred to as 'bad cholesterol'. HDL helps in the removal of excessive cholesterol from the body through the liver. Those who have high levels of HDL, that is, over 45 mg, have a reduced risk of a heart attack. Normal levels of HDL for men are between 36-45 mg and in women, 40-60 mg. Women, in general, have higher HDL cholesterol levels and are, therefore, relatively protected from heart attacks, at least until the age of 50.

HDL Cholesterol Levels & Coronary Heart Disease[1]

HDL Level	Percentage Developing Heart Disease	
	Men	Women
< 25 mg	18	*
25-34	10	16
35-44	10	5
45-54	5	5
55-64	6	4
65-74	3	1
> 75	0	2

* Only four women were in this category; none developed coronary heart disease.

It has been noted that even if the total cholesterol is well within the normal limit of below 200 mg, a person may still have low levels of HDL cholesterol. Dr M. Miller and his colleagues from Johns Hopkins University Hospital in Baltimore, USA, studied a group of 1,000 patients who had already undergone a coronary angiography. It was found that 288 of these patients had normal cholesterol levels. It was of

---

1. 'Framingham Heart Study', Exam 11, as reported by T. Gordon et al. in *American Journal of Medicine* 62 (1977): 707-714.

great interest to note that as many as 67% of men and 80% of women with proven CHD on angiography, had low levels of HDL cholesterol (less than 35 mg in men and less than 45 mg in women). All these men and women had normal levels of total blood cholesterol. Based on their findings, the physicians suggested that a low HDL cholesterol is strongly associated with increased incidence of heart disease. Several other studies have also shown the need for HDL cholesterol estimation especially in the high risk population.

You should consider yourself in the high risk category if:

   You are a man above the age of 45.
   You have a family history of CHD.
   You are a cigarette smoker.
   You have high blood pressure or diabetes.
   You are overweight.

LDL—The 'Bad' Cholesterol: LDL is synthesized in the liver from VLDL. According to the American National Cholesterol Education Programme recommendations, the LDL level should not exceed more than 130 mg. If your LDL is over 160 mg, you are considered to be in the high risk category; LDL levels between 130-159 mg suggest that you are in the borderline risk category.

It has been recommended that all adults over the age of twenty years must, at least, know their total cholesterol levels. Testing for HDL and LDL is recommended for all persons with cholesterol levels of over 200 mg. Although total cholesterol is not affected by meals, for HDL and LDL testing, the person must fast for at least twelve hours prior to the test. In general, this thorough analysis includes results of total cholesterol, HDL cholesterol, LDL cholesterol and triglycerides as well. Since one single reading may not always give you true results, it may become necessary to have two or three different measurements at an interval of 2-4 weeks and take an average of all these readings if there are any doubts about the first set of results.

Ratio of Total Cholesterol to HDL

As stated earlier, it is now being increasingly accepted that the presence of a low HDL level is as dangerous as the presence of a high LDL or high total cholesterol level for the heart.

While a high total cholesterol usually means that there is an associated high LDL level since most of the cholesterol is carried as LDL, the total cholesterol does not really give a true picture of total HDL concentration. For example, a total cholesterol of 240 mg usually corresponds to an LDL level of 160 mg; while a total cholesterol of 200 mg corresponds to 130 mg of LDL. Yet someone with a cholesterol level of 199 mg (within normal limits) may have a significantly lower amount of HDL. 'A low HDL level puts a patient at a high risk of heart attack,' says Dr H. Robert Superko, director of Stanford Lipid Research Clinic.

Indians commonly have HDL levels between 35-38 mg. The exact cause for lower HDL levels in Indians is not quite clear. However, lower HDL levels do put Indians at a higher risk of heart disease. Women, for example, tend to have 10-20% higher values of HDL, and are therefore better protected from heart disease than men.

Rather than a direct measurement of HDL alone, it has been suggested that the ratio of total cholesterol to HDL is more important in determining the risk of heart disease. Let us look at the ratio system from the following examples:

Example. If your cholesterol is 200 mg and your HDL is 40 mg, your ratio will be:

$$\frac{\text{Total cholesterol [200]}}{\text{HDL cholesterol [40]}} = 5$$

Example. If your total cholesterol is 200 and your HDL is 50 mg, your ratio will be:

$$\frac{\text{Total cholesterol [200]}}{\text{HDL cholesterol [50]}} = 4$$

Example. If your total cholesterol is 240 mg and your HDL is 40 mg, your ratio will be:

$$\frac{\text{Total cholesterol [240]}}{\text{HDL cholesterol [40]}} = 6$$

A person with a ratio of 4.5 or lower is considered at a lower risk of heart attack; the higher the ratio, the greater the risk. Clearly, the lower ratio can result only if your HDL is higher and/or the total cholesterol is lower. A person with a ratio of 4 has more heart protection than someone with a ratio of 5.

A small percentage of adults may have a total cholesterol that is close to the desirable level of 200 mg and yet, because of low HDL values, that is, less than 30 mg, may have a high ratio of over 6. These adults are definitely at a greater risk of heart disease.

Based on these observations, some cholesterol experts strongly believe that if you have a history of premature heart disease in your family or if you have other risk factors such as smoking, diabetes, lack of exercise, obesity, high stress, then you must have your HDL level checked, despite having normal cholesterol levels of below 200 mg. All those who have a cholesterol level of over 200 mg, do routinely need further blood testing for HDL, LDL and triglyceride estimation.

Over 70% of heart attack patients have a ratio of more than 5. Dogs and rabbits have almost no heart disease and would you believe that their ratio is approximately 1.5! A newborn child has a ratio of 2 but with advancing years of life, your ratio starts rising. Dr William Castelli, the director of the Framingham Heart Study, suggests that people with a high ratio, because of their low HDL levels, must do everything possible to raise their HDL levels.

5

Measuring Cholesterol

Comment is free but facts are sacred.

CHARLES P. SCOTT

Your cholesterol level is not a fixed number at all times. Several factors including the day-to-day changes in your diet, stress level, and even the time of the day and the weather have been reported to influence your cholesterol results. Several medical conditions and use of medication can also alter the blood cholesterol. Furthermore, different techniques of measurement of cholesterol have also been noted to give different results with the same blood sample. Let us look at some of these factors more closely.

Variability in Testing

Biological Factors: An interesting study entitled 'Day-to-Day Variability of Cholesterol, Triglyceride and HDL' was reported by Dr Bookstein and her colleagues and was published in the well-known medical journal, *Archives of Internal Medicine*, in August, 1990. Blood was tested on three different occasions on Monday, Wednesday and Friday of the same week in fifty-one volunteers.

Significant day-to-day variability was noted as below in three separate blood samples:

Day-to-Day Varibility*

Cholesterol	=	5% variability
Triglyceride	=	20% variability
HDL	=	10% variability
LDL	=	8% variability

* Archives of Internal Medicine (August, 1990).

As a result of their observation, the authors recommended that if an individual's blood cholesterol results were not absolutely satisfactory, then the person required up to three separate testings on three different days. Biological fluctuations, unrelated to age and sex, could be responsible for variations in results. It has been suggested that an average of these readings should become the basis for finding out whether there are high or normal lipid levels. The term lipid includes cholesterol and all of its types, that is, HDL, LDL, and triglycerides.

Variations in Laboratories: In another study, 20 employees of a hospital in Virginia, USA, had their blood samples drawn after a 12-14 hour fast on four consecutive Monday mornings. Samples were tested, both at the local hospital laboratory and at a private laboratory nearby. Interestingly, 10-20% variations in the results were noted between the two laboratories.

Currently, random cholesterol testing, which means testing cholesterol only on one occasion, is not considered sufficient by most experts. A 10-20% variability may result in falsely classifying an individual into a different risk category. While it may give a false sense of security to some people, it may cause unnecessary fear in others. A good example would be someone who is found to have a cholesterol of 205 mg, which is borderline high, in one reading alone; yet, his average of three different readings may be only 195 mg, which is normal.

It is, however, important to understand that 5 to 10% variation is quite common in the field of laboratory testing and occurs in other areas of blood testing as well.

Variation in Measuring Techniques and Equipment:
Another factor is the variation in the laboratory techniques. In the United States today, in many shopping malls, portable analysers are used for quick cholesterol checks. Signs like 'CHOLESTEROL KILLS' or 'TAKE THE TEST THAT COULD SAVE YOUR LIFE', are commonly displayed by these public cholesterol screeners. Although these portable machines are capable of producing satisfactory results, inaccuracies are common because of the temperature and humidity fluctuation. Movement and vibrations can also easily upset the fine tuning of these analysers. Since all treatment decisions are based on actual cholesterol numbers, getting the right test results is crucial.

In 1985 more studies were conducted to check the cholesterol results from different laboratories. The American College of Pathologists sent the same blood specimen samples to 5,000 different laboratories. Laboratories using the Dupont method reported a cholesterol between 222-270 mg on the same sample. A laboratory using the Technicon SMAC method reported results between 250-294 mg, and a laboratory using a third technique by Beekman Astra reported values between 267-397 mg[1]. The true result as determined by the top-notch reference laboratory in Atlanta gave a result of 262 mg. Standards used for calibration of instruments and controls used to monitor results have been blamed for this wide variation. During the past three years, better standardization techniques have made a significant difference in the wide fluctuation of results from different laboratories. However, in many countries, the problem of standardization of equipment still continues and requires closer attention by healthcare officials and regulators.

---

1. The Dupont method, the Technicon SMAC method and the Beekman Astra method use the same specimen of blood. However, since the technique employed and the machine used is different in each case, some variations in the results creep in. These variations can be put into perspective by tallying the test results with the normal values associated with each technique.

Factors that Commonly Affect Blood Cholesterol Readings

Exercise: Regular exercise leads to weight control, while lack of it results in obesity, which is a cause of high cholesterol.

Smoking: Nicotine leads to clogging of the arteries.

Stress level: High stress leads to a build-up of athero-sclerotic deposits.

Position changes before blood testing: A change from lying down to sitting up may raise blood cholesterol because of increased protein in the blood.

Seasonal variations: Cholesterol tends to be 5-8% higher in winter than in summer.

Change in body weight: If you have recently lost weight, your cholesterol is likely to be lower.

Blood-drawing techniques: Your results will be higher if the tourniquet has been applied too tightly or the fingers have been squeezed hard during blood drawing. Cholesterol is bound with blood protein, and during squeezing, the extra protein that is collected in the blood sample will result in a falsely high cholesterol value.

I strongly suggest that if your first cholesterol result is between 190-210 mg, you must have three different readings from blood taken on three different days. Take an average of all these three readings. If the average comes out to be over 200 mg, it is certainly high.

Cholesterol Level during Pregnancy

Cholesterol increases during pregnancy. During the last weeks of pregnancy, cholesterol may be 40-45% higher than the non-pregnancy state.

Cholesterol Level after a Heart Attack

Having a heart attack is a major form of stress, and any stressful condition will lead to a rise in the cholesterol level. This is why the cholesterol values of a heart attack patient are not considered to be very reliable. It takes about three months before a person is considered to reach his/her base level. Although everyone is very eager to know his cholesterol results, one should wait for 10-12 weeks following the heart attack.

Cholesterol Level in Children

Are children's coronary arteries equally at risk of being clogged by excessive fat and cholesterol? This has been a subject of great interest for all parents, physicians and research scientists.

A twelve-member panel of experts in the United States recently prepared a consensus report for the National Cholesterol Education Programme (NCEP). Without any doubt, the panel of experts agreed that children's coronary arteries are equally at risk of damage and blockage over the years if their cholesterol level remains high. In general, the blood cholesterol of children is 10-20% lower than that of adults. The panel of experts classified children into three categories:

Cholesterol Levels in Children

< 170 mg	Acceptable
170-199 mg	Borderline high
> 200 mg	Definitely high

Dr Kurt Gold of the University of California studied 1,077 children between the ages of 2-20 years. The results challenged those who seemed to believe that high cholesterol is a problem limited to adults. Eight per cent of children in this study were found to have a cholesterol level of over 200 mg. Almost half of these children had a family history of high cholesterol. My own belief about excessive television watching and junk food consumption by children was confirmed by this study: 53% of these children with high cholesterol were found to watch 2 or more hours of television per day; some spending as many as 4 hours watching television, were noted to have much higher cholesterol values.

Lack of physical activity, and consumption of food containing high fat and cholesterol was clearly the reason for high blood cholesterol in these children.

In a letter to the Editor of *The New York Times* on October 11, 1989, Dr E.L. Wynder MD, President of the American Health Foundation, urged the need for early cholesterol checking of all children. He even suggested that if a child was noted to have high blood cholesterol, his/her parents should also be checked for high cholesterol levels. In his words: 'Our ability to make an impact on heart disease tomorrow depends on what we do as parents, physicians, health educators and food industrial leaders today.'

According to a report in the 'News from the World of Medicine' in a recent *Reader's Digest* issue, fourteen institutions around America studied 1,800 people between the ages of 15-34 years, who had died in accidents or from other violent causes. Their post-mortem results confirmed the belief that high cholesterol was likely to start showing in the form of clogged arteries at an early age. Another large study was directed by Dr G. Barenson in the United States. Twelve thousand children were studied for 18 years, and it was noted that children with high cholesterol had fatty deposits in their arteries even at the young age of 2 to 3 years. Based on his findings, Dr Barenson also strongly argued that all children must be screened for high cholesterol, and this was the only way to eliminate the threat of heart disease in later years. Dr Richard Garcia from the world-renowned Cleveland Clinic, in Ohio, USA, shares the same thought. Atherosclerosis of coronary arteries starts well before adult life. We know that families with high cholesterol have high rates of heart disease; it is important, therefore, that both the children and the adults undergo blood cholesterol checks.

Even if there are varied opinions regarding the routine cholesterol checking of all children, cholesterol check-ups are definitely indicated for all those children, in whose case, one or both parents have a history of heart disease, or those who are already known to have high cholesterol. In any case, children who are overweight, or happen to be diabetic or hypertensive must have their cholesterol checked.

In the words of Dr Ronald Laurer, the chairman of the Panel of Experts who developed the recommendations for cholesterol screening in children for NCEP in America : 'It becomes the responsibility of the physician treating the adult heart patient to make sure that the patient's children or grandchildren are screened for possible cholesterol or high cholesterol levels.' Children with high cholesterol levels require appropriate advice and close supervision by their parents and physicians. Eating more fruits and vegetables, grains and cereals, and restriction of fatty foods is important. Through frequent monitoring of blood cholesterol results, you can ensure that your child is spared from the disaster of an early heart attack even when he is only 30-35 years old. Remember, it is never too early to start a heart attack prevention programme!

Cholesterol Level in Older People

Heart disease is the leading cause of death in people over the age of 60 years; since cholesterol level rises gradually with ageing, higher cholesterol levels are far more common in old age. The National Centre for Health Statistics in the US studied the total cholesterol levels of thousands of men between the ages of 20-74 years. The following was the estimated prevalence of dangerously high blood cholesterol (over 240 mg) in men:

High Cholestrol Levels in Men

Age	High Cholesterol (Over 240 mg*)
20-24 years	6.2 %
25-34	15.3 %
35-44	27.9 %
45-54	36.9 %
55-64	36.8 %
65-74	31.7 %

* Data based on survey carried out by the National Centre for Health Statistics, USA.

Blood cholesterol levels in old age are subjected to several interacting factors including dietary changes due to loss of teeth and altered sense of smell and taste, alteration in the cholesterol metabolism, and the effects of multiple co-existing medical problems and medication. However, the precise reason for a rise in cholesterol with ageing remains a mystery. Maybe a higher amount of cholesterol is necessary for ageing cells. Cholesterol is an important component of the cell membrane which contains as much as 95% of cellular cholesterol. It has been suggested that the ageing body cells slowly lose their ability to synthesize the cholesterol, and yet, to maintain their proper function, these require a certain amount of cholesterol. Perhaps the blood cholesterol rises at the expense of the poor cholesterol content of the cells.

Checking blood cholesterol in all adults is a considerably large commitment even for rich nations like the United States. The goal of screening is yet to be accomplished even for all those in the age range of 20-60 years. Since most cholesterol studies primarily included men between the ages of 20-60 years, some critics have wondered whether cholesterol lowering can cut down the death rate in older people as well. While the American National Heart, Lung and Blood Institute is currently studying the role of cholesterol reduction in people between the ages of 60-78 years, several reports have already confirmed the high incidence of heart disease in older people with high cholesterol levels. In a study from France, Drs Forette, Tortrat and Wolmark have reported that high cholesterol values are frequent in older women, and if over 270 mg, they are significantly associated with a high rate of heart disease. Therefore they have argued that all women between the ages of 60-80 years must be treated if their cholesterol levels are over 270 mg.

In a recent report published in the *Journal of the American Medical Association*, Drs Benfante and Reed from Honolulu clearly demonstrated that high blood cholesterol was an independent predictor of heart disease even in old age and, therefore, required appropriate attention. This study involved

40

1,480 men all over the age of 65 years: those with high cholesterol levels were noted to be at 60-70% greater risk of suffering a heart attack as compared to older men with normal cholesterol levels. There is little doubt that older people stand to gain from keeping their cholesterol levels low. The famous Framingham Heart Study from Boston has also shown clear advantages of keeping the cholesterol level within normal range for all older adults; lower HDL and higher LDL levels were also noted to result in an increased rate of heart disease. The Framingham Study confirmed that reducing total cholesterol from 285 to 200 mg decreased the risk of heart disease by 33% in people in the age group of 65-74 years, and 23% in 75-84 year-olds.

There have been more reports confirming the benefits of low cholesterol in old age. In a recent annual conference of The American Heart Association, Dr Trudy Bush and her colleagues from Johns Hopkins University Hospital in Baltimore presented some convincing results from their own study. Three hundred and eighty-two white men, all above the age of 65, were studied for a period of over 8 years. Among 43 of them who died during this period, the total and LDL cholesterol levels were noted to be very high. There was an approximately 8% increased risk of death due to heart disease for every 10 mg increase in cholesterol. Compared to those with LDL cholesterol of less than 140 mg, there were almost twice the number of deaths in those with LDL cholesterol of 160 mg and over.

Dr Rubin and his associates from San Francisco published the results of their own study in December 1990 in the *Annals of Internal Medicine,* confirming the fact that reducing cholesterol in old age can lower the risk of heart disease. They studied a total of 2,746 men, all aged between 60-79 years. All of them were observed for over 10 years. Altogether, 260 men died of heart disease during this period. Those with cholesterol levels in the top 25% category had a 50% higher death rate as compared to those with levels in the lower 75% category. Their message, therefore, was clear: the higher the cholesterol, the higher are the chances of death due to heart disease even in old age.

The earlier controversy and doubts regarding the role of cholesterol in causing heart disease in old age is almost over. People over the age of 60 years, just like younger adults, must know about their cholesterol and other risk factors for heart disease. A Los Angeles research project recently tried to study the effects of dietary reduction of cholesterol in older people with high blood cholesterol. Older men, 846 in number, were divided into two groups: a control group that continued with its usual diet, and the other group that was given a low fat and low cholesterol diet. After a period of 8 years of observation, the researchers reported that only 66 people taking low fat and low cholesterol diets suffered from heart attacks or strokes as compared to 96 people consuming the usual diet.

The conclusion from all these studies is certainly very important for a country like India. The Western public might continue to demand more scientific evidence to show that cholesterol reduction is of some value in people over the age of 75 years. This situation applies more to populations in countries like the United States, Canada, Japan and England where people are already living up to the age of 75 to 80 years, and scientists are currently looking for ways to extend their lifespan even beyond this age. In contrast with an average lifespan of 75 years in these countries, the average lifespan in India is about 60 years. So the most important question for Indians has to be: how can we, in the first place, stop the premature deaths of millions of our people between the ages of 40-55 years because of heart disease? In Western countries, for example, the majority of heart patients are between the ages of 60-75 years. With appropriate medical help and self-discipline, they usually manage to live for an extra 10-20 years despite the presence of heart disease. An average heart patient in India, unfortunately, is at a great disadvantage. With little awareness of heart disease and its prevention, and lack of appropriate medical facilities, most patients contracting heart disease at the age of 42 or 48 die within 3-5 years.

Thus we see that there is a substantial amount of evidence that cholesterol reduction can prevent heart disease at all ages, including old age. I would strongly urge that you do everything possible to reduce your cholesterol level, and, thus, cut down your risk of a heart attack even if you are in your 60s or 70s. If you have already lived up to the age of around 60 years without heart disease, wouldn't you like to live for many more years without this dreadful disease?

6

Causes of Heart Attack

Of all the ailments which may blow out life's little candle, heart disease is the chief.

Although heart attack or a coronary thrombosis is a sudden event, the catastrophic event itself is an outcome of coronary artery disease (CAD) that usually takes years to develop. With advancing years of life, the blood vessels tend to lose their elasticity. The hardening and the narrowing of the arteries with deposition of cholesterol and fat (atherosclerosis) in the wall of the coronary arteries interferes with the blood flow. The decrease in the blood supply to the heart commonly leads to angina, the chest pain that arises when the heart muscle is temporarily deprived of sufficient oxygen. A complete blockage of the blood supply to the heart due to the complete blockage of the artery presents itself as a heart attack. While in the vast majority of cases, CAD is the underlying problem for a heart attack, in rare cases, a spasm or sudden constriction of the coronary artery may lead to a heart attack.

Atherosclerosis: A Prime Cause

All arteries are pliable and flexible. A typical artery is made up of three different layers: the intima, media and adventitia. The intima is the innermost layer and has a smooth surface. The smoothness of the intima ensures the continuous flow of blood. Deposits of fat and cholesterol in the intima lead to progressive narrowing and occlusion of the artery. This blockage and degeneration of the arteries due to the build-up of fatty acids is called atherosclerosis. If there is atherosclerosis in the coronary arteries, it may cause a heart attack.

Although heart attacks are rare before the age of 30 years, the process of atherosclerosis surprisingly starts at a much earlier age. Deposits of fat and cholesterol in the intima result in the appearance of fatty streaks. Most people, unfortunately, have fatty streaks in their coronary arteries by the age of 20 years. Fatty streaks slowly increase in size and result in raised areas called fibrous plaques. Over the years the plaques keep increasing in size. The plaques may rupture— and with progressive and repeated bleeding, ulceration, thrombosis and calcification, the blockage of the arteries continues over the years. This process itself is a slow and gradual one. It may take several years—between 10-20 years—for the fibrous plaques and a significant blockage to develop.

A minor degree of blockage may not really interfere with the blood flow to the heart and, hence, remain recognized. It is only when the blockage is severe enough to reduce the blood supply to the heart that a person experiences symptoms. During periods of exercise, the heart demands more blood and oxygen supply. With a rapid heart rate and an increased need for the blood supply, the narrowed artery simply does not allow sufficient blood flow to the heart. Under these circumstances the person commonly experiences chest pain and shortness of breath, which is called an angina attack. Often the person has to slow down and take rest. The need for blood supply diminishes and the pain settles since the partial blockage of the artery does allow some blood to pass through to the heart. Unfortunately, in most cases, the process of atherosclerosis and plaque formation continues, and the

1.

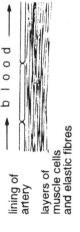

lining of artery

layers of muscle cells and elastic fibres

Normal artery wall.

2.

blood cells rich in cholesterol

muscle cells and elastic fibres

lining

fatty streak

Cholesterol-rich blood cells work their way through the smooth lining to form the fatty streak.

3.

blood particles form a scab on top of damaged lining

growth hormone released by blood particles causes muscle cells to proliferate

cholesterol-rich cells and free cholesterol

Development of atherosclerotic deposit.

4.

fibrous cap to deposit

cholesterol-rich area infiltrated by muscle cells and fibres

Completion of fibrous cholesterol-rich atherosclerotic deposit.

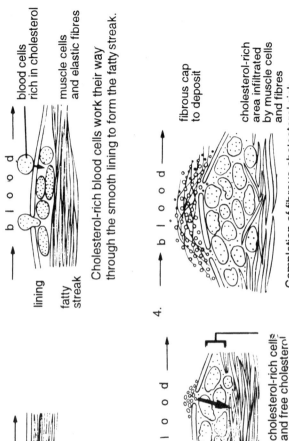

partial blockage then turns into a complete blockage, resulting in a heart attack.

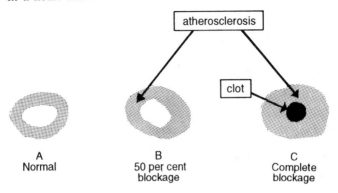

Cross-section of three coronary arteries. (A) A normal coronary artery with a completely open lumen. (B) An abnormal coronary artery whose lumen is blocked over 50 per cent by atherosclerosis. (C) An abnormal coronary artery whose lumen became completely blocked when a clot formed on top of the atherosclerotic plaque, leading to a heart attack and death.

Studies on Atherosclerosis: One of the earliest studies that helped our understanding of atherosclerosis was done by William Enos, Robert Holmes and James Bayer from the US military in 1955. They examined the coronary arteries of young soldiers in their early 20s, who were killed in the Korean War. It soon became clear that the atherosclerotic changes in the coronary arteries commence many years before the actual event of the heart attack. Dr Jack P. Strong, professor and head of the Department of Pathology, Louisiana State University School of Medicine, New Orleans, USA, reported the results of some very interesting studies in 1958. Through his studies he was able to show that all subjects aged 3 years or older had, at least, some amount of fatty streaks; fibrous plaques were noted to be present around the age of 10; and a significant increase in the size of these plaques was found to occur around the age of 30. Further studies by several researchers have confirmed the progressive nature of the process of atherosclerosis. Most authorities believe that changes due to atherosclerosis start in the coronary arteries at least 20 years before the day of the heart attack. Dr Strong, who has been conducting research in the field of atherosclerosis for over 30 years, concludes that: 'Fatty streaks are rare in coronary arteries before the age of 10, but are more frequent between the ages of 10-20, and are present in over 90% of people after the age of 20. Fibrous plaques are more frequent between 20-30 years; by the age of 40, fibrous plaques are present in most people.

Studies of atherosclerosis have been carried out in many countries around the world. An International Atherosclerosis Project (IAP) has studied the problem in 14 different countries. For example, atherosclerosis has been noted to be more pronounced in people from the United States and Norway as compared to Mexico and Japan. It has been shown that the risk factors like high cholesterol and high blood pressure are the reasons for the higher prevalence of atherosclerosis and heart disease in many countries. A well-known study from Oslo—the Oslo study—looked into the lifestyle and risk factors in more than 16,000 men. It was quite clear that the higher mean values of serum cholesterol, triglycerides and blood pressure in the Oslo population were strongly correlated with the increased degree of atherosclerotic plaques in the Oslo population as compared to the Japanese.

The relationship of plaque formation and high cholesterol has been extensively studied in recent years. It has been found that in monkeys and rabbits, raising the blood cholesterol level can lead to fatty streaks and plaque formation. There is no doubt that chances of early and accelerated atherosclerosis are high unless cholesterol is lowered.

Blood Clots in the Coronary Artery

The blood is made up of red cells, white cells and other small cells called platelets. Normally the blood is in a fluid state and continues to flow without any interruption. When and if the blood comes in contact with a broken surface—for example, a ruptured plaque within a wall of a coronary artery— several chemical changes occur which lead to a clot formation. This is a local reaction to bleeding. A similar situation exists when there is a small cut on your finger. When a clot occurs in the coronary artery, it is really dangerous for the heart. The clot may lead to a complete blockage of the artery and cause a heart attack. It is only because of the dangers and the damages caused by a clot that physicians want to dissolve a clot as soon as possible. The sooner the clot is dissolved, the easier it is for the blood supply to be resumed.

7

Heart Attack: Warning Symptoms

*Before thirty, men seek disease; after thirty, diseases
seek men.*

CHINESE PROVERB

CHD has a wide spectrum of presentation. Patients may
suffer from angina or have a sudden heart attack without
any previous symptoms.

Angina: Someone who has angina is troubled by chest pain
on exertion. The chest pain is usually in the form of a heavy
weight or constriction in the central part of the chest. The
pain may radiate to the left arm, jaw, back, neck, or even the
lower chest. Shortness of breath is also a common feature of
angina. Anginal pain, however, is only transitory and usually
lasts between one to fifteen minutes.

Anginal pain is typically relieved by resting or taking a
glyceryl trinitrate (GTN) tablet. If you suffer from angina
you might wonder what kind of course the disease may take.
It is interesting to note that not all patients with angina will
get heart attacks in the near future. You may, in fact, stop
getting anginal pain if your atherosclerosis is made to regress
through substantial reduction of risk factors. In some patients
the disease progresses really slowly.

In a study in England, 200 patients were observed for

several years. The results of the study showed that 25% became pain free; 27% had occasional anginal pain which was controlled with GTN tablets; 6% became severely disabled with frequent pain; and 45% died over the 25-year period of observation with heart attacks or heart failure.

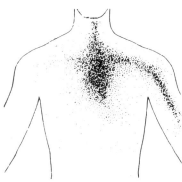

Radiation of angina pain.

Other Symptoms: Someone with CHD may have a sudden heart attack with or without a previous history of angina. Although the precise diagnosis of a heart attack requires an examination by an experienced physician, it is important not to dismiss the symptoms of a heart attack. Unfortunately, too many people just assume that their pain is related to 'indigestion' due to overeating or some unusual food item and, therefore, they even postpone a visit to their doctor. The consequences may be disastrous since, if not recognized at an early stage, a patient with a heart attack may have serious irregular heart beats, or develop heart failure and die suddenly.

Common symptoms of a heart attack include sudden, severe chest pain which may come in the form of a sense of tightness, constriction or heaviness in the central chest area. The pain may be crushing or bursting and is often continuous. It may last for a few minutes, then ease off, but may return within minutes. The pain usually spreads to the left arm but may also be felt in the jaw, neck, teeth or back. In general, the pain is severe and longer in duration as compared to anginal pain. Chest pain may also be associated with shortness of breath, nausea and vomiting, dizziness, sweating and pallor. In a mild heart attack, the person may be able to walk to his physician, and the distress, pain or 'indigestion' experienced

51

by the patient during the heart attack may even have subsided by that time. In a moderately severe heart attack, the degree of chest pain and the severity of illness is much more serious.

Generally speaking, the first 24-48 hours of heart attack are considered the most dangerous as far as the outcome of the heart attack is considered. Most early deaths result from the associated burst of irregular heartbeats that arise from the damaged part of the heart.

Silent Ischaemia: The 'No' Warning Heart Attack

Most people have some idea that during a heart attack a person has severe central chest pain and may have cold sweats, shortness of breath, and a feeling of nausea and vomiting. Yet, in recent years, a new problem of 'silent' heart attack has been recognized and discussed in medical literature. The term 'silent myocardial ischaemia' is used when the body's warning system has altered and an individual patient fails to experience the typical chest pain of angina or heart attack. Both the patient as well as the physician may remain unaware of the problem. Sometimes the condition is diagnosed only when an ECG confirms the presence of a recent or an old heart attack. Why some people have typical chest pain while others do not have any pain with the same degree of ischaemia and atherosclerosis remains unclear. It is possible that some individuals have a higher pain threshold than others.

A recent study of 105 men aged 40-50 years from Norway concluded that up to 4% of these men had the problem of silent ischaemia. Studies have also been done on US air force crews and in apparently, healthy people at Yale University. Based on several studies, it is estimated that approximately 3 to 10% of the adult population over the age of 50 years may suffer from the problem of silent ischaemia.

Though it may take several years for the lay public to learn more about the problem of silent ischaemia, the problem is really a serious one; many victims of silent heart attack may be candidates for sudden death. In people over the age of 60, for example, up to 50% of heart attacks may actually be painless. An older person may have a few symptoms in the absence of severe chest pain, including some shortness of breath, tiredness and lethargy, and the ECG and blood tests may show definite signs of a heart attack. Silent myocardial ischaemia has also been noted to be a major problem in diabetic patients who often have dysfunction of nerve conduction and pain sensation. Similarly, in silent heart attack, the anginal pain that classically comes on due to exertion may really be absent, that is, there may be an actual episode of diminished blood supply to the heart muscle, and yet, the patient may not experience any significant chest pain. In the words of Dr Peter F. Cohn, the renowned New York cardiologist: 'The number of individuals affected by silent heart attack is so large that it is no longer a subject of academic interest; it has really become a major public health problem as well as a challenge to physicians and cardiologists.'

Newer studies during the past fifteen years, including exercise-stress tests and ambulatory monitoring of the rhythm of the heart, have convinced physicians that millions of adults have the problem of silent CHD. Dr Cohn himself has concluded from ambulatory ECG monitoring, that as many as 75-80% ischaemic attacks are associated with little or no pain. Every now and then you hear about somebody who was never known to have any heart disease and died all of a sudden. Why so? Newer techniques for the detection of silent ischaemia are suggesting that the vast majority of these people suffer from silent ischaemia of the heart. In the United States alone, between 350,000-400,000 adults die suddenly each year without any previous diagnosis of heart disease; post-mortem reports show that almost all of them suffered from extensive CHD.

Sometimes adults who are, otherwise, not accustomed to physical exercise, become overenthusiastic about 'Keep Fit' exercises and overexert themselves. Due to pre-existing atherosclerosis, these adults are highly vulnerable to a sudden heart attack and death. This is why all adults over the age o

35 years, with previously sedentary habits, must consult their physician before joining any exercise programme. Patients who have had an actual 'standard' heart attack with chest pain, and so on, may also start experiencing episodes of silent myocardial ischaemia. Cardiac ischaemic episodes, whether painful or not, are a definite threat to the normal functioning of the heart. Patients with episodes of silent myocardial ischaemia are at least three to five times more prone to dying suddenly.

Every Chest Pain Is Not a Heart Attack

Every pain in the chest is not, however, due to a heart attack or angina. A dull ache or sharp, stabbing pain in the area of the heart or left breast is often experienced by neurotic persons. It may be accompanied by palpitations, fatigue and short breath. Overexertion or strenuous work may also cause a person to have a pain in the region of his heart or behind the sternum. Abdominal upsets, an ulcer in the duodenum or stomach, stones in the gall-bladder, inflammation of the pancreas, and even appendicitis may appear akin to a heart attack.

Pain in the chest can occur due to any of several reasons. It is advisable, therefore, to conduct a thorough physical examination of the patient. Lab testing, including an electrocardiogram (ECG) and blood tests will be required to ascertain whether a patient has suffered a heart attack or is suffering from some other ailment.

The imminent danger of CHD cannot be ignored. Checking of blood cholesterol levels and taking the necessary precautions to prevent/control its increase and a timely check-up should take top priority on every individual's agenda.

8

Heart Attack: Are You at Risk?

*Disease is very old, and nothing about it has changed.
It is we who change, as we learn to recognize what
was formerly imperceptible.*

JEAN MARTIN CHARCOT

High blood cholesterol has come to be recognized as a major risk factor in causing heart attacks. Today, at least in the United States, one can hardly find a newspaper or watch a television programme without any reference to the problem of high cholesterol. Although always suspected to be a significant cause, there was continuing controversy regarding the precise role of high cholesterol in causing CHD until 15-20 years ago. However, the controversy has now been settled beyond any doubt. Multiple studies, both in laboratories and in large population groups from several countries, have confirmed that high cholesterol does play a significant role in causing early and premature atherosclerosis and heart disease. The higher the cholesterol level, the greater the problem. What we considered normal only a few years ago is no longer accepted as a desirable level of cholesterol. It has also been clearly noted that the incidence of CHD is higher in countries where fat and cholesterol intake is high; nations with lower dietary intake of fat and cholesterol have a lower percentage of people with CHD.

It is interesting to note, for example, that the average

cholesterol level for adults in Finland and Russia is 30-50 mg higher than that of the adults in Italy, Greece or Japan. It is no wonder that the rate of CHD is fairly high in Finland and Russia. In the United States, over 50% of the adult population has a high cholesterol level of over 200 mg. A level below 200 mg is desirable.

It has been confirmed that the incidence of heart disease starts rising once the cholesterol rises over 150 mg, but there is a significant rise in the incidence of CHD once the cholesterol crosses the limit of 200 mg. After that, for every 1% rise in the cholesterol level, the chances of developing CHD increase by 2%. In other words, if you happen to have high cholesterol and can successfully reduce your cholesterol by even 1%, you can reduce your risk by 2%. Let us say your cholesterol level is 250 mg: if you bring it down by 20%, that is, reduce the cholesterol by 50 mg to 200 mg, you can expect a risk reduction of CHD by 40%. Such is the strong connection between high cholesterol and heart disease. Even though many of these studies have tended to include men, women also are noted to have a higher incidence of CHD if their cholesterol levels are high.

The attitude of the general public as well as the medical community regarding the role of high cholesterol in CHD has changed dramatically over the past eight years. For example, a 1983 survey by the National Institute of Health, USA, suggested that only 39% of physicians and 64% of the general public strongly believed that blood cholesterol reduction had a significant effect on heart disease. The publication of recent cholesterol reports and the launching of the National Cholesterol Education Programme have made a significant impact on the attitude and beliefs of every American.

Today, there is hardly anyone who has any doubt about the strong relationship between high cholesterol and heart disease. As far as medical evidence is concerned, there is no more controversy as to the beneficial effect of lowering cholesterol levels. The benefits of new knowledge can be reaped only if people are determined and consistent about lowering their cholesterol levels. The first step lies in knowing your own cholesterol levels.

Cholesterol Levels: Comparing Your Own Risk

Total Cholesterol Level			
Age	Low Risk	Average Risk	High Risk
20-29 yrs	150-169 mg	170-200 mg	over 200 mg
30-39	155-174	175-200	over 200
40-49	160-179	180-200	over 200
50 and over	170-189	190-200	over 200

LDL Cholesterol Level			
Age	Low Risk	Average Risk	High Risk
20-29 yrs	90-109 mg	110-130 mg	over 130 mg
30-39	95-114	115-130	over 130
40-49	100-119	120-130	over 130
50 and over	105-124	125-130	over 130

HDL Cholesterol Level			
Age	Low Risk	Average Risk	High Risk
20-29 yrs	46-60 mg	40-45 mg	30-39 mg
30-39	46-60	40-45	30-39
40-49	46-55	36-45	25-35
50 and over	46-55	36-45	25-35

During the past thirty years, it has become increasingly clear that heart attacks can be predicted with a sufficient degree of confidence in a given person, based on the presence or the absence of several factors like high blood pressure and blood cholesterol, smoking habits, family history, stress level, physical activity and exercise level, and the presence of co-existing diseases like diabetes mellitus. In the words of Dr Isadore Rosenfeld, clinical professor of medicine, Cornell Medical College, New York, USA:

Heart Attack: Assessing Your Risk

The following questionnaire can help you determine your own risk of heart attack:

Answer the following 14 questions. Response H is indicative of high risk, M means medium risk and L stands for low risk. Answer each question as H, M or L, and at the end of the questionnaire count the total number of H, M or L responses:

1. Your age:

    over 55 years .... H ☐
    between 45-55 years .... M ☐
    below 45 years .... L ☐

2. If one or more of your close family members has had heart disease:

    before age 45 .... H ☐
    between ages 45-55 .... M ☐
    after age 55 .... L ☐

3. If one or more of your close family members has had a stroke:

    before age 45 .... H ☐
    between ages 45-55 .... M ☐
    after age 55 .... L ☐

4. If one or more of your family members has had diabetes mellitus:

    before age 45 .... H ☐
    between ages 45-55 .... M ☐
    after age 55 .... L ☐

5. If your total cholesterol level is:

    240 mg or over .... H ☐
    200-239 mg .... M ☐
    less than 200 mg .... L ☐

6. If your LDL or bad cholesterol level is:

    160 mg or over .... H ☐
    130-159 mg .... M ☐
    less than 130 mg .... L ☐

7. If HDL or good cholesterol level is:

    less than 35 mg (for men)
    less than 40 mg (for women)   H ☐
    between 35-45 mg (for men)
    40-50 mg (for women)   M ☐
    over 45 mg (for men)
    over 50 mg (for women)   L ☐

8. If your triglyceride level is:

over 300 mg	H	☐
200-300 mg	M	☐
less than 200 mg	L	☐

9. If your blood pressure is:

over 160/95 mm	H	☐
120-149/80-90 mm	M	☐
100-120/65-80 mm	L	☐

10. If your body weight is:

8 or more kilograms above normal	H	☐
4-8 kg above normal	M	☐
1-4 kg above normal	L	☐

11. If you smoke:

more than 10 cigarettes a day	H	☐
5-10 cigarettes per day	M	☐
no cigarettes (non-smoker)	L	☐

12. If you consume alcohol:

more than 14 drinks a week	H	☐
7- 14 drinks per week	M	☐
less than 7 drinks per week	L	☐

13. If you exercise for at least 20 minutes:

0-1 times per week	H	☐
2-3 times per week	M	☐
4-7 times per week	L	☐

14. If you estimate your stress level to be:

Very high most of the time	H	☐
Medium most of the time	M	☐
Low most of time	L	☐

Now add up all your responses.

High Risk: Seven or more high (H) responses or five high responses along with five medium (M) responses strongly suggest a high risk of heart attack within the next 5-10 years. The more the low (L) responses, the lower is your risk for heart attack.

A scoring system like this cannot always be absolutely flawless. However, the cause and effect relationship of these risk factors has been repeatedly tested and reported to be true in many scientific studies around the world.

High blood cholesterol, high blood pressure and smoking are three major risk factors for heart disease. Your risk of heart attack is eight times more if you have two of these three problems. With all three risk factors, you are at least 20 times more likely to get a heart attack.

In simple terms, based on our current knowledge, you can easily calculate whether your own chances of getting a heart attack are high, medium or even low.

Are Indians More Vulnerable to Heart Attacks?

For many decades, CHD has been more common in the West as compared to the East or the Far-East. Countries like Japan, China, Taiwan and Korea have been reporting a much lower incidence of CHD as compared to Europe and North America. However, with increasing industrialization, the incidence of CHD is consistently rising even in countries that previously had a lower incidence of CHD. It is important to recognize that simply being of oriental extraction, that is, Japanese or Chinese, does not provide any immunity against CHD.

Several recent reports have confirmed that the incidence of heart attacks has been on the rise in India. It is common to see middle-aged persons suffering, not only from heart disease, but also from high blood pressure and diabetes, particularly, in the upper and middle class categories. People in their 20s and 30s too continue to watch the disability and death of their seniors due to heart disease, and yet, do little to reduce the risk factors for themselves. Indian immigrants in England, South Africa, Fiji and the West Indies have been reported to have a higher incidence of heart disease when compared to other ethnic groups. *The Lancet*, the world-famous British medical weekly, in its editorial of June 7, 1986, referred to the problem of high incidence of CHD in Indians: 'Despite their great cultural and geographical diversity, overseas Indians, wherever they are, appear to have a high mortality rate from CHD in comparison with their compatriots of other ethnic origin. It is estimated that male Indians in America are at least 3-5 times more at risk of developing heart disease.

You may very well ask as to why Indians should be at a particularly high risk of CHD. There are many reasons and some of these are as follows:

High Dietary Fat and Cholesterol Intake: In the United States, during the past 20 years, consumption of animal fat and oils has dropped by 45%. While the Japanese consume the lowest amount of fat, taking only 9% of total calories from all types of fat and only 3% from animal fat, Indians — both in India and outside India — continue to consume a high amount of fat in the form of *desi ghee*, coconut oil, and so on. The Chinese and the Japanese seem to have better and healthier dietary habits. In China, food derived from plant sources such as tofu[1] and vegetables continue to be consumed in large quantities. As a result of these dietary habits, even with modernization and increasing stress levels, lower levels of fat and cholesterol consumption have helped keep the incidence of heart disease low in China.

Smoking: It is by now well established that giving up smoking can significantly reduce the death rate due to CHD. Many Indians have failed to recognize and understand the importance of not smoking. While many people in developed countries have stopped smoking, Indians continue to smoke in large numbers. It is interesting to note that during the past 20 years, tobacco use has gone down by 30% in the United States, whereas, it has shown a consistent increase in India. Approximately 50 million Americans have stopped smoking in the past 25 years. Unless we can significantly reduce the consumption of tobacco in India, we will continue to see an increasing death rate due to heart disease.

---

1. A curd made from mashed soya beans.

High Blood Pressure: The incidence of high blood pressure or hypertension is fairly high in India; millions of Indians suffer from hypertension. Hypertension, at least in the early stages, does not show any symptoms. Unfortunately, many Indians have no idea about their own blood pressure levels. It is not only the illiterate masses, but well-educated Indians who have little information about their own blood pressure. To most of them a disease exists only if they have some significant symptoms or disability. Problems like high cholesterol or high blood pressure that are usually not associated with any symptoms till late, are unfortunately not recognized as significant problems by most Indians.

Lack of Exercise: Only less than 5% of Indians do physical exercise daily. Low educational levels, with associated lack of awareness, may be the underlying reason for leading a sedentary lifestyle. This causes a higher percentage of affluent Indians to have excessive body weight. Obesity itself increases the risk of heart disease. Obese people also have a higher incidence of diabetes mellitus, hypertension and high cholesterol levels.

Genetics: Several medical reports have suggested that Indians have a high incidence of genetically determined fat and cholesterol abnormalities. For example, Indians tend to have high levels of triglycerides and LDL or bad cholesterol, and low levels of HDL or good cholesterol. Drs Enas and Thomas, two Indian physicians from the United States, have reported that South Indians tend to have a high incidence of familial hyperlipidemia, that is, a high level of fat in the blood, with high levels of VLDL or bad cholesterol and low levels of HDL—both increasing the risk of heart disease. An average Japanese has a much higher level of HDL, approximately 55 mg; the average Indian has a level of 35 mg; and the Caucasian-American has a level of 45 mg. Thus, undoubtedly, the Japanese are best protected from heart attacks as compared to both an average American and an average Indian.

Dr Thomas recently reported the results of a comparison of Indian physicians living in the United States with US-born physicians of similar ages. Three interesting findings were noted:

1. Indians had a highly significant elevation of triglyceride levels (174 versus 86 mg).

2. Indians had higher levels of total cholesterol (196 mg versus 177 mg).

3. Indians had lower levels of HDL (36 mg versus 40 mg).

All the above findings can increase the risk of heart disease in any population.

Furthermore, Indians have been reported to have smaller coronary arteries. Hence, even smaller deposits of fat and cholesterol may produce larger obstructions in the coronary arteries. This makes coronary bypass surgery somewhat more difficult, and the results are less than optimal in Indians. But does it all mean that we have already lost the battle against heart disease? Certainly not! If many developed countries can demonstrate a significant drop in the death rate of their populations due to heart disease, India can do the same. In fact, Indians would be expected to make changes in their lifestyle by practicing techniques like yoga and meditation, and turning vegetarian. The role of the right food in maintaining health has been known to ancient Indian medicine for thousands of years. The link between high cholesterol and high incidence of heart disease is no longer a matter of debate, and it is up to you to take steps to reduce your cholesterol and eliminate your high risk of heart disease!

Are Women at a Lesser Risk?

For many years, a misconception prevailed that women were not vulnerable to heart disease. This has proved to be a myth. Each year, in the United States alone, approximately 275,000 women die due to heart disease, accounting for 50% of the 550,000 deaths each year. While fewer women have heart attacks in younger years, it is after the age of 55 that women become equally at risk of getting heart disease as men.

According to Dr A.B. Mehta, Chief of Cardiology, Sion Hospital and Consultant Cardiologist, Jaslok and Breach Candy Hospitals: 'The incidence of CHD is eight times that of men as compared to women in the reproductive phase. From 45 to 60 years, the male-female ratio is 2:1, and above 60 years, it is equal.'

Role of Estrogen in Lowering Heart Disease: The female hormone, estrogen, that is secreted by the female reproductive organs up to the age of menopause, that is, between 45-50 years, is thought to raise the amount of HDL in the blood and lower the amount of LDL. HDL helps in getting rid of the extra cholesterol of the body through the liver and thus provides protection against heart disease in women up to the age of menopause. However, with the disappearance of estrogen after menopause, this protective hormone is secreted only in very small amounts and, therefore, there is an increase in the rate of heart attack after the age of 50 years.

Neglect of Health Care in Women: Even in an advanced country like the United States, a recent study of approximately 5,000 heart attack victims showed that while 26% of men received costly, life-saving, blood-clot-dissolving treatment for heart attacks, only 14% of women with similar heart attacks received such treatment. There have been several other reports confirming that although women sustain identical cardiac disabilities, they are less likely to be treated as aggressively as men. As a result of some of these disturbing findings, the US Congress has now ordered health care agencies to devote more energy and resources towards a better understanding and study of heart disease in women.

Health care of women has been traditionally neglected by society, particularly in countries like India and China, where having sons has always been considered more prestigious than having daughters. It remains a fact that women with many diseases, including heart disease, continue to receive less attention and inferior quality of care by their family members in the vast majority of Indian families even today. At times, the symptoms of heart disease have even been wrongly attributed to psychological depression in women.

Effect of Contraceptive Pills: As discussed before, the beneficial cardiac effect of estrogen secretion in fertile years in women has been well recognized. Hormones in the form of oral contraceptive pills have been used by millions of women in their reproductive years. An interesting question has been raised as to whether oral contraceptives provide any extra protection against heart disease. Extensive studies have, however, shown that taking estrogen in the form of oral contraceptive pills does not provide any extra cardiovascular benefit to women. This is because the quantity of estrogen in the pill is too small to produce a perceptible effect on the heart.

During the past 20 years, at least nine major studies have confirmed that women do benefit from a cholesterol-lowering programme. Women with a total cholesterol of over 200 mg are considered to be at a high risk of developing heart disease just like men.

The old adage, 'Prevention is better than cure' is worth its weight in gold in safeguarding one's health. Recognising one's risk factors by being completely honest with oneself may well be the first step towards improving health. If you have identified your problem areas with a view to taking constructive action in erasing them, delve further to gain a better understanding of these health risks.

PART II
Causes of High Blood Cholesterol

9

Heredity: A Risk Factor

The joys of parents are secret, and so are their griefs and fears.

FRANCIS BACON

The presence of heart disease in the family, in one or both parents or grandparents, does increase your own risk of heart disease. You are two to five times more likely to develop CHD if both your parents have been the victims of heart disease. Moreover, if your parents were unfortunate enough to get a heart attack, for example, before the age of fifty years, you are also at a greater risk of getting a heart attack before you are fifty years old. Our genes control, to some extent, our health and disease pattern as well as the lifespan. Risk factors like high blood pressure, diabetes and obesity that are strongly associated with increased rate of heart disease, also tend to run in the family. Hereditary traits do have a considerable influence in matters of life and death. Also, it is important to remember that families often tend to share the same pattern of smoking, exercise or lack of it, and eating habits.

Interesting studies were done in Finland, a country where coronary heart disease incidence is one of the highest in the world. A study of 211 men with a family history of heart disease was conducted: 50 had heart attacks, 55 died of heart disease and 53 were noted to have angina.

In the remaining 53 individuals where no obvious CHD was noted, the prevalence of medical conditions was studied further. Surprisingly, in these adults with a positive family history of heart disease, high blood cholesterol was noted to be twice as common, and high blood pressure, thrice more common as compared to adults from the families with no history of CHD.

In California, scientists have successfully identified genetic markers signalling an increased risk of CHD and high blood pressure. In one project, 400 patients with definite CHD were studied and compared with 150 healthy persons of a similar age and sex. Curiously, irrespective of the cholesterol levels in these two groups, people with CHD were noted to have specific changes in their genes. A special gene coding for a protein called apolipoprotein was noted. Although a lot more research is needed to precisely detect these changes in the genes, it is becoming quite clear that even without the presence of high blood pressure and high cholesterol, a person with a positive family history of heart disease is at a greater risk of developing similar problems. Genetic tests that can pinpoint the increased risk of heart disease in a particular person are likely to be available before the end of this century.

Dr Diane Becker of the Johns Hopkins University Medical School has reported that premature heart disease in brothers and sisters of the same family is quite common. Her research has suggested that if a family member had a heart attack before the age of 55 years, the sisters would be twice more likely to get a heart attack and the brothers, 10-12 times more likely to be the victims of a heart attack.

Since family history of heart disease increases the cardiovascular risk, the American Academy of Pediatrics strongly recommends an early detection and monitoring of cholesterol in children. Dr Peter Kwiterovich, Chief of Lipid Research at Johns Hopkins University Medical School, suggests that if the cholesterol is high in parents, it is a very good idea to test the children's cholesterol as well.

Genetical Lipoprotein Disorders: Besides dietary problems, there are a number of cholesterol and lipoprotein abnormalities that tend to run in the same families. If the cholesterol problem has a genetic basis, simple dietary changes may just not be enough to control these lipid abnormalities.

It has been reported that Indians tend to have more of the genetic problems that can cause abnormally high cholesterol. There are several genetical lipoprotein disorders with some-what difficult names. Some of the important ones are as below:

➤ Familial combined hyperlipidemia
➤ Heterozygous familial hypercholesterolemia
➤ Polygenic hypercholesterolemia
➤ Familial hypertriglyceridemia
➤ Familial hypoalphalipoproteinemia

'Hyper' finds its origin from a Greek word meaning 'over and beyond'; in medical terminology, it means 'raised' or 'excessive'. Hyperlipidemia, therefore, refers to an excess of fat in the blood; hypercholestrolemia indicates excessive cholesterol in the blood, and so on.

Although you are not expected to remember these scientific terms, it is sufficient to know that familial and genetic cholesterol abnormalities occur in approximately 1-5% of the total population. The knowledge and understanding of these genetically determined cholesterol problems have been acquired only recently. Michael Brown and Joseph Goldstein, the two Nobel prize winners in medicine, have made a major contribution in the field of cholesterol metabolism. The production, clearance and metabolism of cholesterol is quite a complex process. Thousands of receptors are involved in this process. Dysfunction of cholesterol receptor sites on the cells and enzymes may cause abnormally high levels of cholesterol and triglycerides, and raise your risk of heart disease.

The detailed description of all the genetically determined

cholesterol problems is beyond the scope of this book, yet it is important for you to understand that as a result of these genetic disorders, one or more of the following problems may arise:

- Total cholesterol may become high.
- LDL, the bad cholesterol, may become high.
- Triglyceride level may become high.
- HDL, the good cholesterol, may become low.

Unfortunately, if you have inherited any genetic disorder, you may not be completely successful in reducing your cholesterol level.

10

Stress: A Contributory Factor

When two do the same thing, it is never quite the same thing.

PUBLIUS SYRUS

Most people find it difficult to define stress, yet they experience it often. In general terms, stress can be defined as an excessive demand on physical and mental energy, often leading to anxiety, anger, distress, fear, irritability and frustration. This causes an increase in the secretions of pituitary, adrenal and thyroid hormones, and angiotension secretion from the kidneys. All these lead to a rise in the cholesterol level as well as rise in blood pressure, which ultimately result in an increase of fat deposition in the arteries (atherosclerosis), and also coronary heart disease.If stress is left unresolved, the build-up of atherosclerotic deposits increases and the chances of getting a heart attack are enhanced.

There are many situations that can cause stress. Dr Thomas Holmes and Richard Rahe from Washington University Medical School studied a large group of people and developed a scaling system resulting from various stressful events. The death of a spouse was given a score of 100 degrees of stress. The point system as listed on the following pages reflects stress in relative terms only.

Are You under Stress?[1]

Life Stresses	Point Value of Stress
1. Death of spouse	100
2. Divorce	73
3. Marital separation from mate	65
4. Detention in jail or other institution	63
5. Death of a close family member	63
6. Major personal injury or illness	53
7. Marriage	50
8. Being fired at work	47
9. Marital reconciliation with mate	45
10. Retirement from work	45
11. Major change in health or behaviour of a family member	44
12. Pregnancy	40
13. Sexual difficulties	39
14. Gaining a new family member, e.g. through birth, adoption, or older person moving in, etc.	39
15. Major personal readjustment, e.g. merger, reorganisation, bankruptcy, etc.	39
16. Major change in financial state, e.g. a lot worse off or lot better off than usual	38
17. Death of a close friend	37
18. Changing to a different line of work	36
19. Major change in the number of arguments with spouse, either a lot more or a lot less than usual, regarding child-rearing, personal habits, etc.	35
20. Taking on a large mortgage for purchasing a home, business, etc.	31
21. Foreclosure on a mortgage or loan	30
22. Major change in responsibilities at work, e.g. promotion, demotion, lateral transfer	29
23. Son or daughter leaving home, e.g. marriage, attending college, etc.	29

1. Holmes T.H. and R.H. Rahe, 'The Social Readjustment Rating Scale', *Journal of Psychosomatic Research II (1967); 213.*

24.	In-law troubles	29
25.	Outstanding personal achievement	28
26.	Wife beginning or ceasing work outside the home	26
27.	Beginning or ceasing formal schooling	26
28.	Major change in living conditions, e.g. building a new home, remodelling, deterioration of home or neighbourhood.	25
29.	Revision of personal habits, dress, manners, association, etc.	24
30.	Troubles with the boss	23
31.	Major change in working hours or conditions	20
32.	Change in residence	20
33.	Changing to a new school	20
34.	Major change in usual type and/or amount of recreation	19
35.	Major change in church activities (a lot more or a lot less than usual)	19
36.	Major change in social activities, e.g. clubs, dancing, movies, visiting, etc.	18
37.	Taking on a large mortgage or loan for purchasing a car, TV, freezer, etc.	17
38.	Major change in sleeping habits (a lot more or a lot less sleep, or change in part of day when asleep)	16
39.	Major change in number of family get-togethers (a lot more or a lot less than usual)	15
40.	Major change in eating habits, that is, a lot more or a lot less food intake or very different meal hours or surroundings	13
41.	Vacation	12
42.	Major festivals, e.g. Diwali, X' mas, etc.	13
43.	Minor violation of the law, e.g. traffic tickets, jaywalking, disturbing the peace, etc.	11

Interpretation

Low stress	:	0-149
Mild stress	:	150-199
Moderate stress	:	200-299
Major stress	:	300 or more

There are three ways of dealing with stress. You can:
❏ try to avoid situations which cause stress;
❏ change your attitude to situations hitherto regarded as stressful and no longer consider them to be so;
❏ divert your mind and learn to relax more to reduce the physical consequences of stress.

Know Your Personality Type

Based on the individual lifestyle, Drs Freedman and Rosenman have classified most people into two distinct categories. The *Type A person*, who is always in a hurry, finds himself short of time and wishes to complete all projects by a certain deadline. On the other hand, the *Type B person*, who is much more relaxed, usually has sufficient patience without a sense of urgency. Some people seem to think that unless you are rushing and trying to do things with definite deadlines *(Type A),* you are not likely to be a successful person. However, some of the top achievers in the world including Presidents Kennedy and Reagan, Mahatma Gandhi and Jawahar Lal Nehru have been judged as having had Type B personalities.

During a meeting with Dr Freedman, on his visit to New York Medical College in 1989, I had an opportunity to ask him about the success and the failure rate of people from *Type A* and *B personalities.* Without any hesitation, he confirmed that a *Type B person* has equal or even better chances of success in life. Since the *Type A person* is always fighting with himself, he is not utilizing all his talents and time in an efficient manner.

What about your own personality type? Are you a *Type A person* or a *Type B person?* You are likely to be a *Type A person* if the following are applicable to you:

- You are constantly planning and thinking of achieving and accomplishing more and more in less and less time. A chronic sense of time urgency is the hallmark of a *Type A personality*.

- You almost always eat, walk and do things as quickly as possible.

- You are impatient with the way most other people do things. For example, you may even want to complete the sentence of the other person. In other words, you feel that people around you are just too slow.

- You find it very difficult and almost impossible to wait in a line in the post office, or get into the bus, or on a train.

- You are constantly trying to save time and may, in fact, try to complete two to three activities together. For example, you may read a newspaper or go through your mail while eating your meals.

- You feel guilty about not doing 'anything' and relaxing for a few hours or days.

- You strongly believe that all your progress has been primarily due to your aggressive personality, and if you change now, you will be left behind.

- You weigh everything in terms of 'numbers'. Your assessment of others as well as yourself is based only on the amount of money earned.

You belong to *Type B personality* if:

- You sincerely appreciate the virtue of patience.

- You integrate the philosophy of 'all work and no play makes Jack a dull boy', that is, you devote enough time to leisure activities in your life.

- You can relax and do nothing for days and still not become angry and feel guilty about being relaxed.

- You maintain a sense of calmness and security at most times.

- You have none of the characteristics of a *Type A personality*.

Remember that to be a *Type A person*, it is not necessary to have all the characteristics described under the *Type A personality*. If you have more than 50 per cent of the features of the *Type A personality*, you are most likely, a *Type A person*. The *Type A personality* traits are counter-productive and harmful for your heart.

It has long been evident that your personality type holds the key to understanding the cause of CHD. Yet, ironically, the very recommendations made by Western cardiologists today to prevent CHD are those that Indians are, increasingly, abandoning.

11

Lifestyle Addictions

*The unfortunate thing about this world is that good
habits are so much easier to give up than bad ones.*
W. SOMERSET MAUGHAM

Habits are not formed overnight and even though most
people are aware that drinking caffeine-containing
beverages, smoking, and consuming alcohol are health issues,
they are drawn towards them for the stimulation they offer.
This chapter takes a close look at the effects of addiction-
forming habits and cautions you against them.

Tea, Coffee and You

Over half the world's population drinks tea, though in
some other parts of the world, coffee is preferred. Both tea
and coffee contain caffeine[1]. Caffeine is perhaps the most
widely used mood elevator in the world. Through its action
on the brain, it decreases fatigue and tiredness and helps the
tired body and brain to work more efficiently, at least, until
its effect wears off. Tea and coffee are not the only two
sources of caffeine. Several soft drinks including Pepsi and
Coca-Cola contain a significant amount of caffeine. Tolerance
and addiction to caffeine builds fairly fast. Just four or five

---

1. An alkaloid drug with stimulant action found in tea leaves
and coffee beans.

days are enough to build tolerance for caffeine, according to Dr George Koob, a behavioral pharmacologist at the Scripps Institute for Research in California.

We know, however, that if taken in excess, caffeine may cause nervousness, anxiety and sleeplessness. Caffeine is no less than a drug in many ways, and one may easily become addicted to it. Those who are addicted may even experience some withdrawal effects in the form of headaches, muscle pain, stiffness and lethargy.

Caffeine and Cholesterol: Scientists and physicians have been interested in the health effects of caffeine for a long time. A controversy has existed for several years as to whether decaffeinated coffee causes less heart disease and cholesterol changes than regular coffee. Recent studies have tried to answer some of these interesting public health issues regarding the relationship of coffee with cholesterol and heart disease.

In the late 1980s, Scandinavian researchers found that coffee made by boiling ground beans was, perhaps, more damaging to the heart than any other type of coffee. The kind of beans that are used for preparing coffee have been said to influence the cholesterol levels. Strongly **flavoured** *rubusta* beans, commonly used for preparing decaffeinated coffee, have been reported to cause high cholesterol levels as compared to mild *arabica* beans, routinely used for regular coffee. A study of 1,130 graduates of Johns Hopkins Medical School revealed that heavy coffee drinkers consuming more than five cups a day, were two to three times more likely to be at risk of heart disease. There have been several other reports suggesting a link of excessive tea and coffee intake to heart disease. A recent study involving 100,000 people from the Kaiser Permanent Health Maintenance Organization in California concluded that there was a slightly higher risk of heart attack in people who drank four or more cups of coffee per day. Several years ago, Stanford University researchers found that middle-aged adults drinking three or more cups of coffee were more likely to have high cholesterol.

The results of a large study from Norway were published in March 1990 in the *British Medical Journal*. This study confirmed the relationship of excessive coffee drinking and increased deaths due to heart disease. An increased number of deaths due to heart disease were significant in this study even if the rise in the cholesterol was not considered in the calculations. A total of 19,398 men and 19,166 women participated in this large study. All the participants were free of heart disease when the study was started. Cholesterol levels were noted to be higher in the coffee drinkers. Those drinking one cup of coffee a day had a mean cholesterol level of 223 mg; those taking three cups of coffee—a level of 237 mg; and those taking nine or more cups had a cholesterol level of 253 mg. A correlation of deaths due to heart disease was noted; the higher the coffee intake, more were the deaths due to coronary heart disease.

Regular versus Decaffeinated Coffee: Caffeine is the chemical present in both tea and coffee that gives the jolt— the stimulation to the brain and the body. Health promoters have argued that tea is, perhaps, a better drink than coffee largely due to its low caffeine content. Through a process of decaffeination, caffeine contents of regular coffee can be reduced significantly. In many parts of the world, both regular and decaffeinated coffee are available as a choice. It is generally assumed that decaffeinated coffee is less harmful to your body. However, as far as the effect on cholesterol is concerned, a recent study has concluded that decaffeinated coffee may have a worse effect on your cholesterol than regular coffee.

From a study done at Stanford Lipid Research Clinic, Dr Superko and his colleagues reported the effects of both regular and decaffeinated coffee on cholesterol levels. The blood cholesterol of 188 healthy middle-aged coffee drinkers was monitored. For the first two months, these volunteers took three to six cups of regular coffee everyday. After two months, half of them were asked to switch to decaffeinated coffee. Blood cholesterol results were monitored in both groups throughout the study period. The results were interesting. Those who had switched to decaffeinated coffee were found to have an approximately 7% higher level of LDL cholesterol—the bad cholesterol.

Caffeine causes a rise in the blood pressure. In one project, Dr Walter Greenberg and David Shapiro from the University of California studied the combined effect of caffeine and stress on blood pressure. Thirty-six male coffee drinkers were given two different doses of caffeine—125 mg and 250 mg. The mean systolic blood pressure, when compared with that of non-coffee drinkers, was noted to be 5 and 7 mm higher in the adults taking 125 mg and 250 mg of coffee, respectively. When given the mental stress of solving an arithmetic exercise, their blood pressure went up by an additional 10-12 mm of mercury. The researchers concluded that the blood pressure of an average person remains high for up to 45 minutes after a cup of coffee, and in someone who is taking 4-6 cups, high blood pressure may last for several hours and cause damage to the vital organs of the body.

Besides raising the blood pressure, excessive caffeine can also cause irregular heartbeats. In a study reported by Dr Scot Harris from the Baylor College of Medicine, Houston, Texas, 31 patients with a previous history of coronary heart disease were shown to have progressively increasing heartbeat irregularities with increasing doses of caffeine. Heartbeats of patients were monitored continuously for up to forty-eight hours. It was noted that even though increasing intake of caffeine correlated with the frequency of irregular heartbeats, some people could just be oversensitive to caffeine, and get irregular heartbeats even with smaller doses of caffeine.

Thus we see that excessive caffeine intake is associated with increased risk of coronary heart disease. Caffeine is well known to cause an increased heart rate, and may even predispose the individual to a variety of heartbeat irregularities, commonly known as cardiac arrhythmias. In recent years caffeine intake has also been found to cause high cholesterol levels. While one or two cups of coffee per day are considered safe, excessive use of caffeine in the form of tea or coffee is certainly not free from harmful effects.

The Perils of Smoking

Many patients with coronary heart disease have been noted to be heavy smokers. Doll and Hill, the famous research scientists from England, showed many years ago, that physicians between the ages of 35-45 years who smoked, were four times more likely to have a heart attack as compared to non-smoking physicians. The Framingham Heart Study similarly confirmed that smoking substantially increased the risk of heart attacks and strokes. More interestingly, from a 26-year-follow-up of the Framingham Heart Study, Dr Philip Wolf and his colleagues found that cigarette smokers who quit smoking can significantly lower their risk of stroke within 2 years and cut down their risk by 50% within 5 years of cessation of smoking.

Not all smokers run the same degree of risk for developing coronary heart disease. Smoking-related risk of heart disease can be classified as: Low (1-4 cigarettes a day); moderate (5-14 cigarettes per day); or high (more than 15 cigarettes per day). Clearly, a person who has been smoking more than 15 cigarettes a day is at a much higher risk than someone smoking only 2-3 cigarettes per day.

The toxic and cancer-causing substances in the smoke cause slow damage to the epitheliums, the inner lining of the trachea and bronchi. Slowly, the lung tissue continues to be damaged, and the capacity of the lungs to expand is limited, causing shortness of breath. Chronic irritation and destruction of the lining of the respiratory system results in cough, phlegm and repeated infections.

Nicotine leads to the clogging of arteries and blood clot formation. The platelets that are important constituents of the blood are damaged by nicotine. Damaged platelets may lead to blood clot formation in the coronary arteries. Nicotine also increases the clotting of the blood by adversely affecting the concentration of fibrinogen, a blood protein that is often noted to be high in smokers.

Smokers also tend to have high levels of the two hormones, adrenaline and non-adrenaline, in their blood. They are responsible for the 'fight or flight' reaction when a person is under extreme stress. An excess of the two catecholamines —adrenaline and non-adrenaline—can increase blood pressure, heart rate and the oxygen demand of the heart. If the stress is relieved by 'fighting or winning away' from a problem, the threat of a heart attack will be alleviated, but if there is no response to the stress, the overexcitement swelling up within the body may result in an outburst when the body faces another stressful situation. The heart muscle may become extremely irritable and start beating irregularly. In fact, when a person gets a heart attack, it is the presence of excessive catecholamines that usually results in a sudden burst of irregular heart beats and death in most cases.

Those who smoke also have a high blood concentration of carbon monoxide. The blood circulating through the narrowed coronary arteries of a smoker is often full of carbon monoxide. For its proper function, the heart requires oxygen. But instead of oxygen, the blood protein or haemoglobin carries the load of carbon monoxide which is no good for the heart or the body tissues. Without the required amount of oxygen, the heart loses its capacity to beat at regular intervals.

Passive Smoking: Inhaling smoke, when you are in the company of smokers, has also been the subject of attention during recent years. It has been determined that with passive smoking, you are exposed to all the dangers that are associated with active smoking. In a recent study report, Dr Anne Berg of the Yale School of Medicine found that fathers who smoked ran the risk of having children with blood and brain cancers. It has been suggested that smoking may even damage the father's sperms.

Cigarettes versus Cigars: Smoking in all forms is harmful.

Studies have confirmed that men who stop smoking cigarettes and switch to cigar smoking run the same degree of risk of heart disease. Many smokers, particularly those who switch to cigars from cigarettes, inhale a sufficient amount of smoke that can cause damage to their heart and lungs.

Smoking and High Cholesterol: Both smoking and high cholesterol levels are definite risk factors for heart disease. In an interesting study published in the *Journal of American Medical Association,* December 19, 1990, researchers reported the results of their observations of the microscopic changes which had taken place in the arteries of 390 males, 15-34 years old, who had died of violent causes. It was noted that those with high blood cholesterol and a high level of smoking had the most significant changes of atherosclerosis in their arteries.

The combined effects of smoking and high cholesterol are extremely harmful to the lining of the arteries. Continued smoking causes early damage to the walls of the arteries, and the added problem of high cholesterol accentuates the deposition of fat and cholesterol in the wall of the arteries. In simple terms, if a person with high cholesterol is a candidate for heart attack in 8-10 years, a person with similarly high levels of cholesterol as well as smoking is likely to get a heart attack in 4-5 years. The message is very clear. If you have a problem of high cholesterol as well as smoking, take care of both problems.

Alcohol Consumption

Moderate drinking has been noted to have beneficial effects on the heart. Only 1-2 drinks per day is considered moderate drinking. Some studies have suggested that moderate alcohol intake may reduce your chance of developing coronary heart disease. An interesting study involving 18 different countries was recently reported in the *British Medical Journal.* The conclusion of the study was that moderate drinkers were somewhat better protected from heart disease. The study included populations from England, the United States, Japan and Australia.

In a project conducted by the American Cancer Society, 276.802 men were studied for 12 years. Researchers found that in men, the relative risk of death from coronary heart disease associated with 1-2 drinks per day was approximately 70 per cent as compared to non-drinkers. In the Framingham Heart Study, moderate drinkers were similarly noted to have a lower risk of death due to heart disease.

In a recent meeting in San Diego, California, Dr Rodney Jackson reported the results from a study of 2,301 New Zealanders, aged 35-64 years, who had no previous history of heart disease. Moderate drinkers were found to have 30-60 per cent reduction in heart attacks. At the 1990 annual convention of the American Osteopathic Association, Dr Alcin Greber, Professor and Chairman of the Department of Internal Medicine at Southeastern University, Health Science Colleges of Osteopathic Medicine, North Miami Beach, Florida, even suggested a daily alcoholic drink for cardiac protection.

You may wonder as to how alcohol protects your heart. The answer has come from the finding of high concentration of HDL, the good cholesterol, in the blood of moderate drinkers. HDL cholesterol helps in removing the excess cholesterol from the body and, therefore, protects the coronary arteries. Alcohol has also been reported to reduce the tendency of blood clotting by lowering the fibrinogen, a protein necessary in clotting, and decreasing the platelet activity. Platelets are an important constituent of blood and if they are less active, the blood does not clot easily.

Heavy drinking over the years has harmful effects on the heart as well as on other organs of the body. It raises the blood cholesterol level.

Addictive habits of any kind are harmful. It is advisable to check their control over you before you become excessively dependent on them. Learn to say 'no'—to push away temptation and take your health in hand!

12

Obesity — A Large Problem

*Excessively corpulent and excessively lean persons
are alike condemnable. A body which is neither too
stout not too lean, but strikes the mean, is the best.*
SUSHRUTA

Obesity or being overweight is a common problem.
Approximately one in three people in the United States
is overweight. With the rapidly increasing middle and upper
class population, the problem of obesity is on the rise in
India as well.

An obese person tends to have high blood pressure, high
blood cholesterol and diabetes mellitus. As confirmed by the
Framingham Heart Study, all these three problems increase
the risk of heart disease. It has also been noted that even in
the absence of high cholesterol and high blood pressure,
obese people are more at risk of coronary heart disease.

Obese people commonly have high blood cholesterol, a
high level of triglycerides and high LDL or bad cholesterol.
In many overweight people, the HDL or good cholesterol
level is low. Obese people often consume high amounts of
fatty foods. Excessive amounts of calories, saturated fat and
cholesterol in such foods are responsible for the high blood
fat levels.

Obese people are also noted to have high blood pressure
in greater numbers. In fact, one piece of important advice

that an obese person with mildly high blood pressure can follow is to lose some weight. In many cases, simply losing some body weight is enough to bring the blood pressure to normal levels. The weight loss in an obese person is also helpful in lowering the blood cholesterol. It is estimated that between 30-40 per cent of hypertensive patients can successfully reduce their blood pressure without requiring drug therapy, if they can successfully lower their body weight by reduced caloric intake and regular physical exercise.

It has also been noted that once an overweight person suffers a heart attack, his chances of death are far more than that of a person who suffers a similar heart attack but has normal body weight. The increased risk of death in obese patients who suffer a heart attack results from excessive blood clot formation and the spread of these clots to different parts of the body, such as the heart, lungs and brain.

Dr Natoobhai Shah, a senior consultant and cardiologist, Bombay Hospital, presented one of the first studies on younger populations aged 40 years and below at the Asian Pacific Congress in Singapore. Shah feels that the profile of predominantly vegetarian patients in this study proved that sedentary lifestyles and obesity were the main factors in CHD.

13

Diseases Which Cause Elevated Cholesterol Levels

All commend patience, but none can endure to suffer.
THOMAS FULLER

It has been found that certain diseases lead to a rise in the blood cholesterol level. This, in turn, can precipitate a heart attack or sudden death. Victims may be unaware of the risk factors relating to such diseases, and by the time they decide to make a serious effort to control the disease, it may be too late!

Diabetes

High cholesterol is a common problem in diabetic patients of all ages. Coronary heart disease is, perhaps, the single most important reason for the death of diabetic patients. In 1927, Joslin, the world-renowned expert in diabetes mellitus, wrote: 'I believe the chief cause of premature development of atherosclerosis in diabetes, except for advancing age, is an excess of fat—an excess of fat in the body which is called obesity, an excess of fat in the diet, and an excess of fat in the blood. With an excess of fat, diabetes begins; and from an excess of fat diabetics die, formerly of coma, and recently of atherosclerosis.' Unfortunately, even though sixty-five years have passed since then, doctors continue to pay insufficient

89

attention to the control of cholesterol and fat in diabetic patients.

Diet and Diabetes: The treatment of diabetes with tablets or insulin injections will work well only if you stick to a sensible diet. Eating food rich in starch and sugar can lead to difficulties in controlling your blood sugar. With poor control of diabetes, you are likely to experience a sense of weakness and tiredness. A high amount of sugar in your blood may cause you to pass excessive urine, both during the day as well as the night. You may start losing weight despite an increased appetite and thirst. Why is this so? The reasons are quite clear. With poor control, your body tissues are not able to utilize the glucose from the blood and provide you with sufficient energy. When blood loaded with sugar passes through your kidneys, the kidneys fail to re-absorb the sugar and thus, your energy is consistently lost in the form of excessive glucose in the urine.

Complications of Diabetes: Patients who have persistently high blood sugar are at risk of many of the common complications of diabetes as listed below:

Angina pectoris due to narrowing of the coronary arteries.

Heart attack due to the blockage of coronary arteries.

Peripheral vascular disease. You may experience pain in the legs when walking. The pain is relieved upon taking rest and thus you are able to walk again before the pain returns. The condition worsens progressively. With effective control of diabetes and blood cholesterol, one can prevent or at least delay this condition for a long time.

Nephropathy—kidney failure.

Neuropathy—nerve damage.

Retinopathy—loss of vision.

Diabetic patients commonly have high levels of triglycerides, a type of fat that has also been considered an independent risk factor for early heart attack. Altogether, a high total cholesterol, with high levels of LDL— the bad cholesterol, and triglycerides, and a low level of HDL— the good cholesterol — all result in an increased risk of heart disease in diabetic patients. Diabetic patients also tend to be overweight. Obesity itself is a separate risk factor for heart disease.

In a report published in July 1989 in the *Journal of American Medical Association*, Dr Michael Stern and his colleagues reported cholesterol results of 460 adult diabetics. Over 40 per cent of them were noted to have cholesterol levels of over 200 mg; an additional 23 per cent had high levels of triglycerides and/or low levels of HDL.

Diabetic patients with poor control have a particularly serious risk of developing heart disease. Poor diabetic control is invariably associated with high cholesterol. The higher the cholesterol, the more the risk of heart disease. Several other risk factors like hypertension and obesity are also far more commonly seen in diabetic patients. Each of these risk factors will further increase the risk of heart attack.

Many diabetic patients and their family members, unfortunately, remain unaware of these risk factors. If a diabetic patient has been consuming excessive fat and cholesterol in the diet, the problems of coronary heart disease can worsen significantly. Our current knowledge of the process of atherosclerosis dictates that diabetic patients must not take high fat diets. Kidney damage itself, commonly present in diabetic patients, may also contribute to high cholesterol levels. Furthermore, drugs like beta-blockers and thiazide diuretics commonly used by diabetics patients may also lead to high blood cholesterol.

High Blood Pressure

It is by now well established that uncontrolled high blood pressure or hypertension significantly increases your risk of coronary heart disease. For example, a 40-year-old man with uncontrolled systolic blood pressure of 196 mm is almost at five times greater risk of stroke or heart attack within the next seven years than one who has normal blood pressure. Dr Roger Williams and his colleagues conducted a study of the families of 15,475 high school students in Utah, USA, and concluded that high blood cholesterol was very common in patients with hypertension.

Furthermore, a greater number of these patients tend to be smokers, diabetics and overweight people. In simple terms, a patient with hypertension is likely to have several risk factors as compared to someone with normal blood pressure. Clearly the more the number of risk factors in one person, the higher are his chances of heart attack. Lipid research clinic studies have also confirmed that cholesterol abnormalities are up to 4.2 times more common in patients with hypertension as compared to adults with normal blood pressure.

In addition to high blood pressure itself, certain drugs like beta-blockers and thiazide diuretics—commonly used in the treatment of hypertension—may also result in high cholesterol levels. Even though a cholesterol of less than 200 mg has been accepted as normal in an adult, in a large scientific study, hypertension patients with a blood cholesterol level of 182 mg and over were found to have a significantly higher rate of heart disease. Reports from the United States and Australia have provided enough evidence that people with high blood pressure ought to be extremely careful about their cholesterol levels.

Both high blood pressure and high cholesterol levels are commonly present in the adult population. Between 15-25 per cent of the adult population in India is estimated to have high blood pressure. Similarly, between 20-30 per cent of all Indian adults are thought to have high cholesterol levels of over 200 mg.

Other Diseases

There are some other diseases besides diabetes and hypertension that may also cause a rise in the blood cholesterol. Some of these diseases are discussed below:

Thyroid Disorders: Thyroxine is a hormone that is produced by the thyroid gland in small quantities. It plays an important role in the body and affects all the body organs.

In the case of thyroxine deficiency that commonly results from an underactive thyroid gland, the body metabolism slows down. This condition is known as *hypothyroidism*. The patient may start gaining weight. The heart, brain and even the digestive system may also adversely affect the blood cholesterol. It is also common to find a high cholesterol reading of 250-350 mg in patients with hypothyroidism.

It has been known for more than fifty years that patients with underactive thyroid glands are more prone to developing coronary heart disease. In recent years, it has been shown that thyroxine deficiency leads to a deficiency of specialized LDL receptors in the body and, therefore, your body cannot easily get rid of an excessive amount of cholesterol. Thyroxine deficiency also causes obesity. High blood cholesterol and obesity are the two most important reasons for high incidence of heart disease in people with an underactive thyroid gland.

On the other hand, patients with an overactive thyroid gland (*hyperthyroidism*) have an increased metabolic rate and tend to have low blood cholesterol levels. In fact, some 25-30 years ago, when accurate and more precise tests for thyroid functioning were not available, abnormal cholesterol level results were often used as an indicator of thyroid gland activity.

Kidney Diseases: At least 50 different types of kidney diseases may result in a syndrome called *Nephrotic Syndrome*. Patients with nephrotic syndrome typically lose a lot of protein in the urine. While a normal person loses less than 100 mg of protein in the urine in 24 hours, a patient with nephrotic syndrome can lose between 5-20 gm of protein per day. As a result of the excessive protein loss due to kidney damage, the blood protein level diminishes. Almost all these patients develop swelling or oedema of the legs and feet. Many nephrotic patients also have high blood pressure. Over 70 per cent of patients have high blood cholesterol, high LDL cholesterol and triglycerides. It is believed that because of low blood protein levels, the liver tends to produce excessive amounts of cholesterol and triglycerides.

Irrespective of the precise mechanism of increased production of cholesterol, a nephrotic patient is at a greater risk of developing coronary heart disease because of persistent high blood cholesterol. Furthermore, because of the excessive swelling of the legs, many of these patients are taking diuretics or 'water pills' that may also contribute to high blood cholesterol levels.

Pancreatic Disease and High Cholesterol: The pancreas is one of the most important glands in the body. Its main role is to secrete insulin and control the blood sugar level. Acute inflammation of the pancreas, called pancreatitis, may cause a high blood cholesterol level. However, such a high blood cholesterol level is not considered to be a real risk factor for heart disease since blood cholesterol returns to a normal level once the pancreatitis is cured—usually within a period of less than ten days.

Armed with proven knowledge that diseases such as diabetes, hypertension, thyroid disorders, and so on lead to a rise in cholesterol levels, the prevention and/or speedy cure of these diseases becomes singularly important. One disease should not be allowed to lead to another and definitely not to one which is far more threatening to life.

14

Drugs which Cause Elevated Cholesterol Levels

Half the modern drugs could well be thrown out of the window, except that the birds might eat them.

MARTIN H. FISCHER

Patients suffering from diseases which require treatment with medication may find themselves in a difficult situation. Many types of medicines have been noted to cause high cholesterol due to their toxic effects.

Diuretics: A group of medicines that make you pass more urine and are frequently used for the treatment of hypertension and heart failure, may increase your cholesterol. Commonly-used diuretics include *chlorthiazide, hydrochlorthiazide* (ESIDREX), *chlorthalidone* (HYTHALTON), *fruesamide* (LASIX), *bumetinide* (BUMET) and *ethacrynic* acid. Besides causing a rise in the total cholesterol, diuretics may also increase LDL and triglyceride levels and lower the HDL level. If your cholesterol is high and you are taking a diuretic, your physician may, either, decide to change the medication altogether or may prefer to reduce the dosage.

Beta-blockers: This is a group of special medication that was first introduced in the early 1970s. Today millions of people are taking beta-blockers for hypertension, angina or heart irregularities. In the past 20 years, beta-blockers have, undoubtedly, saved millions of lives around the world. Yet, like all other medications, beta-blockers have their own side-effects. One of the main problems is that high cholesterol is commonly associated with their use. Commonly used beta-blockers include the following: *propranolol* (INDERAL), *metapropranolol* (METOLAR), *atenolol* (LONOL), *timolol, lebetalol* (NORMADATE), *pindolol* (VISKEN).

Currently almost all the above mentioned beta-blockers are freely available in India. Is there a beta-blocker that is completely free from this problem? Unfortunately, most beta-blockers cause a rise in cholesterol. *Timolol* is perhaps the only exception. Like diuretics, beta-blockers cause a rise in LDL cholesterol and triglycerides, and decrease HDL levels.

Specific Drugs for Hypertension: Apart from beta-blockers and diuretics, other commonly used drugs for high blood pressure may also cause abnormalities in cholesterol or other types of lipoproteins. *Prazosin, captopril* (ACETEN) and *methyl* dopa (ALDOMET) are other commonly used agents prescribed for hypertension that may raise your cholesterol.

Other Medications: Besides drugs used for the treatment of hypertension, angina and heart failure, several other medications have been reported to cause cholesterol disturbances. Some of these are:

- Anabolic steroids
- Androgenic hormones
- Corticosteroids, commonly used for asthma, rheumatoid arthritis and many allergic conditions
- Contraceptive pills

Fortunately not all side-effects are common. It is only through a blood test that you and your doctor can find out whether your cholesterol has been adversely affected by taking a particular medication. If a drug is raising your cholesterol, safer and alternative medications must be used. It is simply no good to have consistently a high blood cholesterol level due to any medication, however effective it may be in controlling hypertension, heart failure or any other disease.

PART III
Lowering Your Cholesterol

15

Dietary Changes

*For extreme diseases, extreme strictness of treatment
is most efficacious.*

HIPPOCRATES

High blood cholesterol and high LDL or bad cholesterol
levels are associated with a high incidence of coronary
heart disease. If blood cholesterol is lowered in such
individuals, their rate of heart attacks goes down significantly.
The famous Framingham Heart Study confirmed that even
with a 10 per cent decrease in the cholesterol level, you can
expect to reduce your risk of heart attack by as much as 20
per cent.

Who Needs Dietary Changes?

As a result of the above information, the National
Cholesterol Education Programme (NCEP) was launched in
the United States a few years ago. According to the NCEP
recommendations, all adults can be classified into three
categories based on their total cholesterol and LDL or bad
cholesterol levels.

NCEP Classification According to Total Blood Cholesterol Level

Level		Assessment
< 200 mg	=	Desirable blood cholesterol.
200-239 mg	=	Borderline high blood cholesterol.
240 mg or >	=	High blood cholesterol.

The NCEP announced practical ways of treating the problem of high cholesterol.

If your cholesterol is:

Below 200 mg: continue with a sensible low fat and low cholesterol diet. Have your cholesterol checked every 3-5 years.

Between 200-239 mg and if you have two other CHD risk factors as given below, but no known CHD: continue with a low fat and low cholesterol diet and have your blood cholesterol checked every year.

Between 200-239 mg and if you have been diagnosed to have CHD levels: have further blood tests for LDL,HDL and triglyceride levels.

240 mg or over: have further blood tests for LDL, HDL and triglyceride levels.

For the above plan of action, the following CHD risk factors were recognized by the NCEP:

1. Male sex
2. Family history of premature CHD
3. Cigarette smoking
4. Hypertension
5. Low HDL-cholesterol level
6. Diabetes mellitus
7. History of definite cerebrovascular or occlusive peripheral vascular disease
8. Severe obesity (30% overweight)

NCEP Classification According to LDL Level

Level		Assessment
< 130 mg	=	Desirable LDL cholesterol
130-159 mg	=	Borderline high risk
160 mg and >	=	High risk

LDL, the bad cholesterol, requires checking only if cholesterol is over 200 mg. It is important to understand that LDL is thought to be the main culprit in causing the process of hardening and narrowing of the coronary arteries. Based on the LDL level alone, the NCEP devised the above classification and recommended the following plan of action:

If your LDL is:

Less than 130 mg and you have no CHD and /or no two or more risk factors: enjoy a normal diet but restrict it to a low fat and cholesterol intake.

Less than 130 mg but you have CHD or two or more risk factors: follow Step-One diet as discussed later.

Between 130-159 mg and you have no CHD and/ or no two or more risk factors: you need treatment with diet alone; LDL must be brought to below 130 mg.

Between 130-159 mg and you have CHD and/or two or more risk factors: you need treatment with diet, drugs or both.

160 mg and over: you need treatment with diet, drugs or both.

Stepwise Approach to Dietary Treatment

Dietary treatment must not be taken lightly. Before a person with high cholesterol begins dietary treatment, it is important that he discusses his complete medical history, family history and any other drugs that he may be taking with his doctor. The goal of the therapy is to lower the total cholesterol to less than 200 mg and LDL cholesterol to below

Two-Step Dietary Therapy
To reduce High Blood Cholesterol Level

Recommended Intake: Step One

Nutrient	
Total fat	< 30% of total calories
Saturated fatty acids	< 10% of total calories
Polyunsaturated fatty acids	Up to 10% of total calories
Monounsaturated fatty acids	10% to 15% of total calories
Cholesterol	< 300 mg/day
Carbohydrates	50% to 60% of total calories
Protein	10% to 20% of total calories
Total calories	To achieve and maintain desirable weight

Recommended Intake: Step Two

Nutrient	
Total fat	< 30% of total calories
Saturated fatty acids	< 7% total calories
Polyunsaturated fatty acids	Up to 10% of total calories
Monounsaturated fatty acids	10% to 15 % of total calories
Cholesterol	< 200 mg/day
Carbohydrates	50% to 60% of total calories
Protein	10% to 20% of total calories
Total calories	To achieve and maintain desirable weight

130 mg. During the treatment, it is not necessary to check the total and LDL levels regularly. If the total cholesterol has gone down below 200 mg, it is more likely that the LDL has declined as well.

Although the dietary changes may sound simple, it is not always easy to change dietary habits. Some people may over-enthusiastically force themselves to go on a strict diet in the first few weeks, but they soon start feeling bored and depressed and may go back to their original food habits. A considerable amount of discussion and encouragement is essential to achieve satisfactory results. Remember, when you decide to change your eating patterns, you are committing yourself to a lifelong change. A simple two-step dietary approach as given in this chapter should be followed.

As you have seen from the given table, the dietary changes are designed to slowly and progressively reduce the intake of saturated fat and cholesterol. Both in the Step-One and Step-Two diets, the total fats must be reduced to less than 30 per cent of the total calories. In the Step-Two diet, the saturated fat is further reduced from less than 10 per cent to less than 7 per cent of the total calories. While the Step-One diet allows you to take up to 300 mg cholesterol per day, the Step-Two diet limits the cholesterol to less than 200 mg per day. Some overenthusiastic patients often wonder if they would do better by completely eliminating the saturated fat and cholesterol. Your body can certainly function well without any saturated fat in your diet. However, severe limitation of fat will surely affect the taste of your food.

It is not always easy to fully understand the amount of calories that different food products contain. Since the success of any dietary programme depends upon a thorough understanding, you need to really discuss this matter with your doctor and a qualified dietician. The Step-One diet must be tried strictly for, at least, three months. It is no use testing the blood cholesterol every one to two weeks. A monthly cholesterol check is sufficient. A falling cholesterol level will not only be great news for you but can also act as a source of encouragement to keep you going.

If after a trial period of three to six months, the Step-One diet has failed to lower the cholesterol, you should switch to the Step-Two diet. The Step-Two diet has even less fat and cholesterol, and is expected to produce better results in lowering the cholesterol. Treatment with medication is required only if the dietary modifications fail to lower the cholesterol even after a period of six to nine months.

16

Fight Free of Fats!

*Animals feed; man eats. Only the man of intellect and
judgement knows how to eat.*

BRILLAT-SAVARIN

Fat adds to the taste of all foods and it is, therefore, not easy to lower the fat contents of the food for most people who become used to a particular type of food. Even in a country like the United States where people are far more literate and educated, the average American takes too much fat in his daily diet. Over the past 30 years, at least 17 major health organizations including the American National Institute of Health and the American Heart Association, as well as the United States Surgeon-General have all repeatedly advised Americans to cut down their intake of fat and cholesterol. Despite all these efforts, in the average American diet, over 37 per cent of all calories are taken in the form of fat. Most health authorities agree that the amount should be cut down to, at least, below 30 per cent. During the past five years, many experts have even advised that the calories from fat should be cut down to less than 25 per cent. Diets containing between 10-15 per cent of fat have been shown to reverse the process of narrowing of the coronary arteries in many heart patients.

Saturated versus Unsaturated Fats

There are two main types of fat— saturated and unsaturated. Fats are made up of glycerol and fatty acids. The composition of fatty acids varies in different fats. In some fatty acids, all the carbon atoms are attached to, or saturated with hydrogen atoms. These are known as saturated fatty acids. If, in a fatty acid, some carbon atoms are not attached to hydrogen atoms, that fatty acid is called unsaturated. If the number of unattached carbon atoms is single, the fatty acid is known as monounsaturated, and if the number of unattached carbon atoms is large, it is known as polyunsaturated. Saturated fat is found mostly in foods of animal origin such as milk, butter, *ghee* and meat. Saturated fat is solid at room temperature. Some vegetable oils like coconut and palm oils are also rich sources of saturated fat. It is the saturated fat that causes the major problem of atherosclerosis and coronary heart disease.

Unsaturated fats are typically found in oils; these fats remain liquid at room temperature. Unsaturated fat may further be divided into the monounsaturated or polyunsaturated type. As compared to saturated fat, both monounsaturated and polyunsaturated fats are much safer for your heart. Limited use of unsaturated fats may, in fact, lower your cholesterol and reduce your chances of heart disease. Food sources of monounsaturated fats are olive, canola and almond oils. Polyunsaturated fats are found in corn, sunflower and fish oils.

A recent study from Holland confirmed the importance of consuming more olive oil which is a monounsaturated fat. Twenty-four men and twenty-four women between the ages of 18-59 were put on two different diets for 36 days. Those consuming a diet rich in olive oil had lower cholesterol levels as compared to those taking a diet rich in saturated fat. In a major article published in the *Journal of American Medical Association* on June 26, 1991, Dr Warren S. Browner and his colleagues suggested that if all Americans restricted their intake of saturated fat and cholesterol, there could be a 15-20 per cent reduction in the death rate due to heart disease.

106

Their best estimate was that dietary restriction of saturated fat from 37 per cent to 30 per cent alone would save approximately 42,000 lives per year. In another published report on June 19, 1987, in the *Journal of American Medical Association*. Dr Paul T. Williams and his colleagues reported (from a study of 76 sedentary middle-aged men aged 30 to 55 years) that increased intake of olive oil also resulted in lowering the blood pressure.

The effects of dietary fat modification on blood cholesterol have also been studied in children. Researchers in Finland studied 36 children aged 8-18 years. Upon reduction of dietary fat from 35 per cent to 24 per cent, there was a 15 per cent reduction in cholesterol. When the children were put back on their original high-saturated-fat diets, their blood cholesterol levels went up to their initial levels.

Resisting Fast Foods

Not only in Western countries but in many developing countries as well, the increasing trend of fast life has resulted in people consuming excessive amounts of fast foods. A noted cardiologist in America recently concluded that the rapid growth in fast food restaurants has almost paralleled the rise in the incidence of heart disease. It is estimated that in the United States, 5 per cent of all adults eat their breakfasts, 20 per cent have their lunches and 16 per cent have their dinners in fast-food restaurants. Altogether over 45 million people visit these restaurants daily. Mr Phil Sokolof, a 67-year-old industrialist, who nearly died from a heart attack some twenty-five years ago, has led a consistent war against the high fat content of fast foods in the United States. As a result of his efforts, famous fast food chains like McDonalds, Burger King and Wendy's have recently decided to cut down saturated fats in hamburgers, French fries and other foods.

The Dangers of *Desi Ghee*

Desi ghee and butter are two prominent examples of saturated fat. It is estimated that while the highest source of saturated fats in the Western diet is red meat, in countries like India, the highest amount of saturated fat is consumed in the form of butter and *ghee*. Many rich and well-to-do people take great pride in consuming pure *desi ghee* in their homes. Some truly wealthy people, unfortunately, still believe that vegetable oils can make them sick, and only visit restaurants where pure *desi ghee* is used for cooking.

Vegetable *ghee*, like Dalda and other brands, requires hydrogenation for converting oils that are normally liquid at room temperature to the vegetable *ghee* that is solid at room temperature. Whereas only 13% of calories in corn oil comes from saturated fatty acids, vegetable *ghee* contains between 25-30% calories from saturated fat. Approximately 65% of the calories in butter come from saturated fat.

A high intake of saturated fat can almost certainly give you a heart attack. Your risk is, of course, much more if you have other additional risk factors. Dr Dean Ornish in California has recently shown that by cutting down the total fat to less than 10 per cent in the diet, many heart patients can even reverse the narrowing of their coronary arteries. You can also help your heart a great deal if you can replace *desi ghee* with cooking oils like groundnut or corn oils.

Facts about Cooking Oils

Both monounsaturated as well as polyunsaturated fats are helpful in reducing blood cholesterol. While most oils are rich sources of unsaturated fats, they also contain some saturated fat. The percentage of monounsaturated, polyunsaturated and saturated fat of different oils is listed in the table overleaf.

The benefits of olive oil have been widely discussed in medical literature during the last five years. Because of the low incidence of heart disease in Mediterranean countries, such as Spain and Italy where olive oil is used extensively, Western scientists became interested in finding out the possible role of olive oil. It soon became clear that olive oil reduces blood cholesterol and, therefore, provides protection for the heart.

Percentage of Saturated and Unsaturated Fat in Different Cooking Oils

Oil	Saturated	Monounsaturated	Polyunsaturated
Almond	9	73	18
Butter	65	30	4
Canola	7	62	31
Coconut	92	6	2
Corn	13	25	62
Cottonseed	27	19	54
Groundnut	18	48	34
Palm	51	39	10
Safflower	9	13	78
Sesame	15	42	43
Soyabean	15	24	61
Sunflower	11	20	69
Olive	14	77	9
Vegetable *ghee*	28	45	27

17

Choosing the Right Foods

Doctors are always working to preserve our health and cooks to destroy it, but the latter are often more successful.

DENIS DIDEROT

S ensible dietary changes can certainly reduce blood cholesterol and the risk of heart attacks. Recommendations about the foods that you should take and those you should avoid are discussed in this chapter.

Fruits and Vegetables: Fruits and vegetables not only abound in vitamins and minerals but also provide plenty of fibre in our daily diet. A high amount of fibre can reduce blood cholesterol and the risk of heart disease.

In India, we are fortunate to have a variety of seasonal vegetables. It is well established that those who consume large amounts of vegetables have a lower risk of developing heart disease. All vegetables tend to be low in calories and, unless fried, have no fat or cholesterol. Therefore, it is not surprising that the best heart specialist would advise you to, at least, double your intake of vegetables if you are serious about reducing your risk of heart disease. However, remember that excessive heating and frying with saturated fat or *desi ghee* can easily neutralize many of the health benefits of fruits and vegetables. Many people just prefer to eat boiled or steamed vegetables. If you must, use only small amounts of cooking oil to fry your vegetables. Adding a lot of *ghee* may add to the taste but your heart will have to pay a price for it.

Due to their lower caloric content, no fat and no cholesterol, oranges and orange juice consumption is great for your heart. Lemon juice too is completely free from fat and cholesterol. Being a rich source of vitamin C and an antioxidant vitamin, lemon juice is a good choice for your heart.

Grapes also have a high vitamin content and lack fat and cholesterol. They are, therefore, excellent for your heart.

Milk, Curd and Yoghurt: Milk is an excellent source of protein, calcium, phosphorus and vitamins. In Western countries, three to four types of milk are freely available. Milk containing 1%, 2% and 4% of fat (whole milk), and skimmed milk without fat are readily available. For the prevention of coronary heart disease, skimmed milk is, of course, ideal. A cup of skimmed milk contains 60 calories as compared to 160 calories contained in wholemilk.

Dairy products including curd and yoghurt are widely used in all countries. In India, many people like to take a regular glass of *lassi*[1] during the summer months. In Western countries, there are varieties of yoghurt made from milk containing between 0-4% fat. Many types of yoghurt also contain fruits and different flavours. Yoghurt consumption has been noted to lower the blood cholesterol. Low fat yoghurt (*lassi* without the butter part of the curd) is, of course, an excellent choice for your heart.

Bread, *Chapati* and Rice: Bread with its different names, including *chapati* or *roti*, has been one of the important foods that is consumed all over the world. Bread, if made with whole grains, contains a lot of fibres which are good for the heart as they lower blood cholesterol. Refined white

---

1. Buttermilk.

111

flour bread does not give you the same advantage. Bread may also be prepared from other grains including corn, guar or soya bean flour. Mixed flours not only add to the taste but also increase the nutritional value of the bread.

The lower the added fat in the bread, the better it is for your heart. In recent years, there has been a substantial increase in the consumption of 'no fat, no cholesterol' breads. While preparing *chapatis* at home, it is wise not to put *ghee*, oil or salt in the flour.

Unrefined or natural brown rice is a rich source of fibre. Rice loses its fibre with refinement. In many countries rice bran products that are rich in fibre are also available.

Fibre-rich Foods: High fibre intake can reduce the chances of coronary heart disease, diabetes mellitus and obesity. High intake of soluble fibre has been found to lower the blood cholesterol by 10-25 per cent. Oat bran is high in soluble fibre which lowers the absorption of cholesterol in your digestive tract. During the past ten years, the use of oat bran has risen enormously in Western countries. *Isapgol*[2], a fibre-rich product widely available in India, has been reported to lower the cholesterol at least 5-8 times more effectively than oat bran. In general, all cereals and grains are rich in fibre and are good for the heart. (See Chapter 20 for a detailed discussion on fibres).

Almonds and Other Nuts: Almonds and all other nuts are rich in fatty acids and protein. However, almonds have a high ratio of monounsaturated fatty acids; consumption of monounsaturated fats can reduce the total cholesterol and LDL, the bad cholesterol. A study conducted in California used natural almond oil as a major source of fat in the diet. After four weeks, it was noted that the total cholesterol had reduced both in men and women. During the study, the other types of fat intake was kept low. Therefore the researchers concluded that the use of almonds had a cholesterol-lowering

---

2. A medicinal plant.

effect. Ten to twenty almonds per day are good for the heart and the body in general.

Besides almonds, walnuts and groundnuts are other types of nuts that merit special mention. Since the vast majority of Indians cannot afford to consume costly walnuts or almonds, peanuts are a good substitute. Groundnut oil is rich in unsaturated fat and is, therefore, much better than *desi ghee* or saturated fat for the heart.

Foods to Avoid

There is a tendency in affluent people to consume more of fat and cholesterol-rich foods. As a result, these people tend to suffer from obesity, diabetes mellitus, high blood cholesterol, high blood pressure and coronary heart disease. The following foods must be avoided as much as possible:

Red Meat: Red meat, typically, includes pork and beef. Excessive use of red meat has been associated with an increased risk of heart disease. Many people in Western countries have reduced their consumption of red meat in recent years because of the high amount of saturated fat and cholesterol it contains. The consumption of red meat must be restricted to only occasional events. Instead, poultry meat may be taken as *tandoori* or barbequed so that little fat is added to it.

Eggs and Cheese: While egg white contains albumin, the protein part of the egg — the eggyolk— contains all the cholesterol. An average-sized egg has between 250-300 mg cholesterol. Since you should limit your cholesterol intake to less than 300 mg per day, taking more than one egg a day is considered to be harmful. Since you may be taking other foods containing cholesterol, even one egg per day may not be desirable. You can discard the yellow part of the egg to reduce your cholesterol intake. A sensible approach to a healthy heart dictates that you take not more than three to four eggs per week.

While the protein and caloric content of cheese make it a desirable food, the high fat and high caloric values of cheese cause problems, particularly for those who are overweight and have high cholesterol levels. In recent years, low-fat cheese has been made available in several countries. That is certainly a better choice.

Coffee, Tea and 'Colas': The excessive use of caffeine can cause high cholesterol levels, anxiety and heart beat irregularities, Not only tea and coffee, but many of the soft drinks including Pepsi and Coca-Cola contain caffeine.

Coconut and Coconut Oil: Each 100 gm of coconut contains 14 gm of fat. Unfortunately, the majority of this fat is saturated. Both coconut and palm oils contain high amounts of saturated fat and should, therefore, be avoided as much as possible. Peanut and saffola oils are better choices.

While choosing a particular food, it is important to think in terms of calories, fat and cholesterol content of the food items.

Amount of Cholesterol in Different Foods

Food	Cholesterol mg per 100 gm	Food	Cholesterol mg per 100 gm
Brain	2000	Beef	70
Egg, whole	550	Fish, steak	70
Kidney	375	Fish, filet	70
Liver	300	Lamb	70
Butter	250	Pork	70
Oysters	200	Cheese spread	65
Lobster	200	Margarine, (2/3 animal fat, 1/3 vegetable)	65
Heart	150	Mutton	65
Prawns/Shrimp	125	Trout, if cooked with additional fat	62
Cheese, Cheddar	100	Chicken	60
Lard and other animal fat	95	Ice-cream	45
Veal	90	Whole milk, 1 cup	34
Milk, dried, whole	85		

114

Cottage cheese, creamed	15	Rice, if no fat is added	0
Mayonnaise, 1 tablespoon	10	Aerated drinks	0
Skimmed milk, 1 cup	5	Almonds	0
Apple Juice	0	Carrots	0
Banana	0	Egg Plant	0
Cashew nuts	0	Potato	0
Egg white	0	Peas	0
Jam, Jelly	0	Cucumber	0
Lentils	0	Spinach	0
Mango	0	Lady Finger	0
Peanuts, roasted	0	Cocunut	0
Sugar	0	Peanuts	0
Vegetables	0	Sugar	0
Vegetable oil	0	Beer	0
Asparagius	0	Whisky/Gin/Vodka/Rum	0
Bean Sprouts (moong)	0	Tea/Coffee	0
Cabbage	0		

18

Fish Lowers Cholesterol

The art of healing comes from nature, not from the physician. Therefore the physician must start from nature, with an open mind.

PARACELSUS

It is well known that heart disease is rare in Eskimos. It is not as if Eskimos do not consume any fat. They do, in fact, eat a lot of raw meat. But they also consume a lot of fish, including seals and whales. In 1994, Hugh Sinclair noted the rarity of heart disease in the Eskimos while working in the Royal Canadian Air Force. Sinclair, along with some Danish investigators, studied a colony of Eskimos from Greenland, who were noted to have a very low incidence of coronary heart disease. Sinclair even transported a deep-frozen seal to Oxford in England. For one hundred days he ate nothing but seal, fish and water . What happened to his blood cholesterol? On this primarily fish diet, his blood became thin and difficult to clot. He also had some bruising and nosebleeding. Soon it became clear from further blood tests that high consumption of fish and fish oils could lower the blood cholesterol levels and delay the clotting of the blood.

In recent years, a number of studies have confirmed that sufficient consumption of fish and fish oils can reduce the likelihood of a heart attack and even death in those who are likely to get a heart attack. Let us look at some interesting results. In a study published in the *American Journal of Cardiology* in November 1990, Dr Rois and his colleagues from the Harvard Medical School reported a significant reduction of LDL and triglycerides (both bad forms of cholesterol) with a fish oil supplementation in the diet. Dr Francois Meyer from Laval University Hospital in Canada has even shown from his study of 107 patients, that eating fish helps in the prevention of narrowing of coronary arteries or re-stenosis in patients who have undergone balloon angioplasty for their heart disease.

A study published in the *Lancet*, the world-renowned weekly British medical magazine, involved 2,000 patients who had already suffered from heart attacks. Half of these patients were advised to eat fish at least twice a week. The results over the next two years were astonishing! Those eating fish were significantly less likely to die from heart attack as compared to those not eating fish.

Other studies have also shown similar results. At the Second International Conference on Preventive Cardiology at Washington in the summer of 1989, Dr Therse Dolecek presented the results from 6,000 men aged 35-57 years. Those consuming the highest amount of fish were noted to have the lowest rate of death due to heart disease. In another case, 852 middle-aged men from Holland were studied for twenty years. Twice the number of deaths due to heart disease were reported in those who ate no fish as compared to those who ate fish, at least, twice a week. Studies in pigs have even shown evidence of reversal of atherosclerosis in those pigs who were fed with cod liver oil for several months. Pigs who were not given the oil were not found to have these benefits.

Omega-3 Fatty Acids

Fish oils are the fats extracted from fish and shellfish, either from their flesh and fatty tissue, or from certain organs such as the liver. These fats differ from animal fats. Though there is a wide variety of fatty acids present in fish oils, two are especially useful in lowering cholesterol: EPA

117

(eicosapentaenoic acid) and DHA (docosahexaenoic acid). EPA and DHA are both polyunsaturated fatty acids.

EPA is a chain of twenty carbons with five areas of unsaturation. Since it has an area of unsaturated carbon atoms at the third position from its tail end, it takes the name of omega-3 ('omega' meaning 'last'). Similarly, since DHA has an unsaturated area at the sixth position from its tail end, it is known as omega-6.

EPA reduces the tendency of the blood cells and platelets to form blood clots. Omega-3 further reduces LDL and increases HDL, thus reducing the chances of narrowing of the blood vessels and protecting the heart from atherosclerosis. Another effect of EPA is a decrease in the production of triglycerides in the liver.

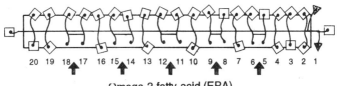

20 19 18 17 16 15 14 13 12 11 10 9 8 7 6 5 4 3 2 1

Omega-3 fatty acid (EPA)

Schematic drawing of an omega-3 fatty acid (EPA). The chain of carbon atoms is depicted by a straight line, to which are attached hydrogen atoms (shown as squares) or oxygen atoms (shown as shaded triangles). The carbons in the chain are numbered, by convention, from the acid end (far right), and the areas of unsaturation are indicated by arrows. The tail end (far left) contains the last, or omega, carbon.

In one study, 20 patients with high cholesterol levels were given salmon fish oil for four weeks. Their blood cholesterol went down by 27 per cent and their triglycerides were reduced by 64 per cent. However, not all types of fish and fish oils have similar cholesterol-lowering effects. While salmon fish can significantly lower the cholesterol, cod liver oil has only a mild cholesterol-lowering effect. The variety of fish that are noted to help in reducing the risk of heart disease through cholesterol lowering, usually live in deep, cold ocean water. Fish containing higher amounts of omega-3 fatty acids are better for your heart.

Apart from the cholesterol-lowering effects, taking fish and fish oil can also reduce your risk of heart attack by altering your blood-clotting mechanism. Studies on normal volunteers and heart disease patients in England and Sweden have confirmed that taking fish and fish oils decreases the clotting of blood. Blood clotting occurs as a result of a favourable change in the action of omega-3 fatty acids on the platelets which are the blood cells directly involved in the blood-clotting process.

Another cardiovascular benefit was reported by Dr. Fordon Margolin and his associates from the Jewish Hospital of Cincinnati in USA. They found that fish oil helped in the reduction of blood pressure. These researchers studied 46 patients with high blood pressure for a period of four months and noted a drop of 12 mm and 5 mm of mercury in the systolic and diastolic blood pressure, respectively—a result of fish oil supplementation.

Thus we see that increased consumption of fish and fish oil can reduce your chances of heart disease. It is, however, essential to select the type of fish that is rich in omega-3 fatty acids. Eating fish two to three times a week is definitely helpful in reducing your risk of heart disease. If you are a vegetarian, you may consider taking fish oil capsules. However, these capsules do not compensate fully for the benefits of actually eating fish. In the United States, the Food and Drug Administration has concluded in favour of eating more fish rather than substituting it with fish oil capsules. In the words of Dr William B. Kannel, professor of medicine and epidemiology at the Boston University Medical School and the founder of the Framingham Heart Study: 'My advice is to eat whole fish rather than fish oil, since you get a meal out of it.'

Fish Containing High Omega-3 Acids

Fish*	Hindi	Tamil	Telegu	Kannada	Oriya	Marathi	Bengali	Gujarati	Malayalam
Herring *Pellona* (Indian) *brachysoma*	Hilsa	—	—	—	Paunia piuce	—	—	—	Kannan Mathi
Mackerel *Rastrelliger Kanagurta*	Bangda	Kumla, Kanan-	Kaman-godechalu gathi	Bangada	—	Bangada	—	—	Aila
Halibut		—							
Sturgeon		—							
Salmon *Polynemus* (Indian) *tetradacylus*	Samon, Mridup	Puzha-kkala aksha, maga Neel Matsya	Budatha	Vameenu, Rawasi	—	Rawas	Gurjowli	—	Bameen
Bluefish									
Sablefish									
Sardines *Sardinella fimbriata*	Charee-addee	Sudai	Kavallu	Pedi, Erabai,	—	Pedwa, Washi	Khaira	—	Chala mathi
Anchovy *Engraulis* (Indian) *mystax*	—	Poruva, Nethal	Poravallu	Manangu	—	Kati	—	—	Manangu

* The zoological names of the fish are given in italics

120

Eel	Sarpa meen	—	Vilangu Kozhi Pambu,	—	—	Vam. Bale	Bam	—	Pambu Meen
Eel (Fresh water)	—	Seram-pambu	—	—	Ahir	—	—	—

Fish Containing Lower Amounts of Omega-3 Fatty Acids

Fish*	Hindi	Tamil	Telegu	Kannada	Oriya	Marathi	Bengali	Gujarati	Malayalam
Catfish *Arius sona*	Ashalk	Mandai kaleru	Tedijella	Mogam-shede	-	Shingala	-	-	Valia etta
Cat Fish (Fresh Water)	-	Keluthi	Jellalu	Shede					Etta
Catfish (Pungas)	Pariaisi	Kovail	-	-	-	-	Pungwas	-	-
Carp	Safari	-	-	-	-	-	-	-	-
Bass	-								-
Perch	Kawaee								-
Haddock	-			-		-			-
Turbot (Indian)	-		-	-		Kuppa	-	-	Sura
Red Snapper	-		-	Kemmasue	-	Tambusa	-	-	-
Sword Fish	Tenga			-		-			-
Rainbow Trout	Trout	-	-	-	-	-	-	-	-
Trout									
Tuna *Thynnus macropterus*	-			-	-	-	-	-	-
Dogfish	-	-	-	-	-	-	-	-	-
Lake Trout	Trout	-	-	-	-	-	-	-	-

* The zoological names of the fish are given in italics

122

19

The Value of Garlic

Because the newer methods of treatment are good, it does not follow that the old ones were bad: for if our honourable and worshipful ancestors had not recovered from their ailments, you and I would not be here today.

CONFUCIUS

Though ancient Indian medicine has recognised the value of garlic for thousands of years, it is only recently that the Western world has become interested in garlic. Garlic is being increasingly accepted as an aid in the prevention of diseases like hypertension, coronary heart disease, blood-clotting disorders, and even cancer. So much so, that in 1990, some fifty scientists and physicians from all over the world gathered in Washington to discuss and share their views about the exact role of garlic in the promotion of health and prevention of disease.

Benefits of Garlic

Garlic contains more than 200 different chemical compounds. The promising findings and possible benefits of garlic have led the prestigious National Cancer Institute of America to devote more than 20 million dollars to the research and study of this substance. In the United States, Dr Robert Lin, the organizer of the First World Congress on Garlic, has emphasized that the medical community must try to understand and utilize the health benefits of garlic. Asians, including the Japanese, Chinese and Indians, have long believed in the medicinal value of garlic and included it in their diet; the use of garlic is comparatively recent in Western countries. In Germany over twenty per cent of the adult population is currently said to be taking garlic pills regularly. However, garlic is best taken in its natural form. Since a lot of people find it difficult to take it raw, it can be chopped finely, or ground and taken with buttermilk, yoghurt or milk. Some of the medical benefits of garlic are as given below:

Blocks Cholesterol Formation in the Liver: In a normal person, between 70-80 per cent of the cholesterol is synthesized in the liver; between 20-30 per cent of blood cholesterol comes from the dietary intake. The sulphur compounds in garlic block the formation of cholesterol in the liver and, thus, the total blood cholesterol level declines. The concentration of bad cholesterol, that is LDL, and triglycerides goes down; the good cholesterol, HDL, is raised. The net effect of all these changes is a reduction in the risk of heart disease. For example, in a study from the University of Wisconsin in the United States, animals fed on garlic were found to have lower levels of LDL cholesterol.

A study conducted by Dr Arun Bordia from the Tagore Medical College in Udaipur, Rajasthan, has clearly established the benefits of garlic. This study was carried out in collaboration with the state of Pennsylvania and the Federal Department of Agriculture in the United States. A total of 432 patients who had already suffered a heart attack were divided into two groups. One group received a daily supplement of garlic juice in milk; the other group did not. The results were revealing! Patients in the group that received garlic juice were noted to have lower blood pressure and lower cholesterol, and had a lesser number of second heart attacks and deaths as compared to adults in the group that received no garlic. In fact, the death rate in the garlic group was approximately 50 per cent as compared to the 'no-garlic' group. Those who took garlic also reported better general health and improved physical and sexual performance. Furthermore, garlic was noted to reduce the incidence of joint pains and asthma as well. Altogether, the results of this study have been very encouraging and favourable for regular garlic use. By virtue of its effects on cholesterol, regular garlic use can significantly reduce your risk of heart attack.

Reduces Tendency of the Blood to Clot: Garlic can reduce the tendency of the blood to clot by blocking the formation of thromboxane, a clotting factor, and lowering the level of fibrinogen, a blood-clotting protein. Blood-clotting disorders are responsible for deep vein thrombosis, pulmonary embolism, stroke and heart attacks. Millions of people die each year due to these problems. It has been claimed that garlic may even be better than aspirin in preventing a blood clot.

Blocks Nitrosamine Formation: Some of the chemicals in garlic have been noted to block the nitrosamine formation in the body. Nitrosamines are thought to cause cancer of the stomach. Cured meats and charred foods are capable of causing more cancers because of excessive formation of nitrosamine. Adults taking regular garlic have been reported to have lower incidence of stomach cancer in countries like China and Italy. The American National Cancer Institute is currently studying approximately 3,000 adults in collaboration with some Chinese scientists. Early studies from the Penn State University have already suggested that garlic can cut down the risk of cancer of the oesophagus, mouth, larynx, stomach and colon.

Possesses Anti-infective Properties: Garlic has been suggested to have anti-infective properties. In Russia, farmers are said to plant garlic among strawberry plants as a defence against destructive insects. In ancient cultures, garlic was worn around the neck to prevent colds. Garlic can potentiate your immune function—the body's power to fight against infection. People who eat garlic regularly are noted to have fewer colds and coughs.

The Western world is becoming increasingly enchanted by the medicinal value of garlic. In California, the Fresh Garlic Association has launched a campaign to increase the consumption of fresh garlic in the United States. In the state of New York, garlic growers have already started to celebrate September 14 of each year as 'Garlic Day'!

The strong pungent smell of garlic is caused by the sulphur in the garlic. It is becoming clear that garlic does not have to be consumed in its raw form to be effective. Some drug companies have successfully eliminated the smell of garlic. Garlic tablets and capsules are being currently used in many countries.

Some Precautions: If taken on an empty stomach, garlic can cause stomach upsets, and even stomach ulcers and blood loss. Some people may find, that like any other food item, they are allergic to garlic. If you think you are allergic to garlic, you must see your doctor before you take any garlic products. Garlic must, in any case, be taken in moderation. Starting with one clove of garlic a day, upto five cloves daily may be taken. Though it is best taken in the morning, due to its strong smell, some may prefer to take it at night.

20

Fibre Helps

In treating a patient, let your first thought be to strengthen his natural vitality.

RHAZES

Fibre is the structural part of fruits, vegetables and grains that cannot be digested by the human body. Fibre is also called bulk or roughage. It was the British surgeon, Dr Denis Burkitt, who first took up the banner of a high-fibre diet in preventing some of the common diseases of this century. In 1970, he reported from Africa that over a twenty-year period of observation, he had rarely seen patients with coronary heart disease, colon cancer and gallstones in Africa, and this could all be due to the high-fibre diet of the Africans.

Research has confirmed that high fibre intake can, substantially, cut down the risk of many common diseases including obesity, diabetes mellitus, gallstones, hypertension, high cholesterol and heart disease. Dietary fibre has, of course, been known to prevent constipation for a long time, but its role in many other conditions has become clear only during the past twenty years.

High Fibre Lowers the Risk of Heart Disease

High fibre intake is associated with low incidence of heart disease. In one study of twenty developed countries, it was noted that populations with a high fibre intake had a lower rate of heart disease. Japan, for example, was noted to have the highest fibre intake and the lowest incidence of CHD. The United States, on the other hand, had the lowest fibre intake and the highest rate of heart disease. Other studies from England and Holland have confirmed that people with the lowest fibre intake have four to five times more CHD than those with the highest fibre intake. It has been suggested that fibre intake may be reducing the incidence of CHD even if the cholesterol lowering is only of a small degree. In one recent study, adults taking approximately 17 gm of soluble fibre were noted to have 13-26 per cent lower cholesterol levels within a few weeks. Numerous medical associations around the world have endorsed the concept of cholesterol lowering through dietary changes as the most important step in the prevention of heart disease.

Types of Fibre

Fibres are of two types: Water-soluble and Water-insoluble.

Water-soluble fibre includes all gums, pectins and mucilages. Water-soluble fibre binds the bile acids in the intestine and, therefore, reduces the cholesterol by reducing the total cholesterol in the body. The liver has to then use more of the circulating cholesterol to manufacture bile acids, since bile

Water-Soluble Fibres

Type	Plant Source	Food source	Action
Pectin	Binds cell wall in plant tissue, giving a gel	Gel in fruit; some vegetables and legumes	Holds water and binds bile acids
Plant gum	Sticky material at point of plant injury	Fruits and vegetables	Water-binding capacity; used as emulsifier
Mucilages	Gelatinous substance similar to plant gum	Guar gum (legumes); plant seeds; part of fruits and vegetables	Influences plasma glucose and insulin levels

Fibre in Your Foods

Fibre in gm per 100 gm of food

Fruits		**Rice, polished**	0.80

Fruits

Apples	1.42
Bananas	3.40
Grapes (white)	0.90
Grape fruit	0.60
Oranges	1.90
Peaches	
(skin included)	2.28
Pears	2.44
Plums	
(skin included	1.52
Strawberries	2.12
Watermelons	1.00

Vegetables

Beans	2.90
Beetroot	3.10
Brocolli tops	3.60
Brussels sprouts	4.22
Cabbage	3.44
Carrots	2.90
Cauliflower	2.10
Cucumber	0.40
Mushrooms	2.50
Okra	3.20
Onions	1.30
Potatoes	3.41
Radish	1.00
Spinach	6.30
Turnips	2.20

Legumes and Lentils

Peas	7.75
Lentils	2.20

Cereals and Wheat products

Oatmeal porridge	7.66

Rice, polished	0.80
Wheat bran	44.00
Wheat flour (100%)	13.51
White flour	3.45

Nuts

Almonds	14.30
Coconuts (fresh)	13.60
Peanuts	7.60
Walnuts	5.20

Non-Vegetable foods

Milk (cow or buffalo)	0
Butter	0
Cheese	0
Beef	0
Pork	0
Mutton	0
Chicken	0
Fish (all types)	0
Lobsters	0
Prawns	0
Oysters	0
Eggs	0
Leak	3.1
Pusley	9.1
Chick Peas	15
Sweet Corn (boiled)	4.7
Appricot (dried, raw)	24
Appricot stewed	8.9
Black currant (raw)	8.7
Dates (dried)	8.7
Figs (dried, raw)	18.5
Prunes (dried, raw)	16.1
Guemes	3.6
Aubergin	2.5

acid bound with soluble fibre, is excreted with the faeces. It is important to remember that only the water-soluble fibre has the capacity to lower the cholesterol.

Water-insoluble fibre is particularly good for digestive disorders including prevention of constipation, diverticular disease and cancer of the colon.

Water-Insoluble Fibres

Type	Plant source	Food source	Action
Cellulose	Chief part of cell wall of plant	Wheat bran and 25% of plant fibre	Speeds up gastrointestinal transit and faecal bulk
Lignin	With cellulose makes up cell wall of plant and the cementing material between cell wall and cell	Vegetables and fruits	May bind bile acids and other materials
Hemicel-lulose	Part of cell wall, less complex than cellulose and easily changed to simple sugar	50-70% of plant fibre of grains and vegetables	Helps relieve constipation

Water-insoluble fibre primarily comprises of lignins, cellulose and hemicellulose that helps in the formation of bulk and, thereby, makes it easy for the stools to travel in the large bowel.

Note : Many food items are rich, both in water-soluble and insoluble fibres.

The Role of *Isapgol* (Psyllium), Oats and Guar Gum

Isapgol or Psyllium has been known and used for centuries in ancient Indian medicine. In recent years, because of its high-soluble fibre content, *Isapgol* has been noted to reduce the cholesterol level. In one study, after an eight-week intake of psyllium, a 15-20 per cent reduction of LDL cholesterol was noted in men with high cholesterol. Other studies have shown similar results.

India is one of the principal producers of *Isapgol. Isapgol* is not expensive and is readily available. Regular *Isapgol* intake can reduce your cholesterol by 10 to 25 per cent.

Oat and Oat Products have been popular in Western countries for a long time. Oatmeal, a grain that has high-soluble fibre, is widely used as a cereal. Although oatmeal, as a **cereal**, has been available for many years in the West, the actual health benefits of oat bran have come to light only recently. In 1977, Dr Anderson, a pioneer researcher, decided to investigate the role of oat bran, the outer part of the oat that contains the most fibre and is not digested by the body. The Quaker Oat Company in USA, in fact, informed Dr Anderson that though they knew all about oatmeal, they had not heard of oat bran. The company referred Dr Anderson to an oat-milling plant. The plant executives informed Dr Anderson that oat bran was a byproduct of milling oat flour and was only used for pet foods. When Dr Anderson received the first shipment of oat bran, he used it on a number of people, including himself. To his great surprise, Dr Anderson's own blood cholesterol declined from 280 mg to 175 mg—a 30% drop on 100 gm of oat bran a day just after 5 weeks! The rest is history! Today, millions of Americans start their day with oat bran breakfasts.

By now there are well over twenty scientific studies confirming that regular use of oatmeal can reduce cholesterol. Oats are, however, not commonly cultivated in India. The Indian answer to oats is *Isapgol. Isapgol* has been shown to be five to eight times more potent in lowering cholesterol. Major cereal-producing companies like Kelloggs in the United States have recently marketed *Isapgol* in the form of breakfast cereals under the brand name of Heartwise.

Guar is a fibre found in legumes, particularly, in their seeds. It contains high-soluble fibre and some Indian companies have even come up with guar tablets. Like oats and *Isapgol*, studies have confirmed that guar gum intake also lowers the cholesterol level. In one study, after two to three months of 13-18 gm of guar gum intake, it was noted that cholesterol was reduced by 15-20 per cent.

Steps to Increase Your Fibre Intake

The recommended adult intake of fibre is 40-50 grams per day. Most adults take less than 50 per cent of the daily recommended allowance. Steps to eat more fibre, as suggested by the Health Education Council of England, and based on exprience of other authorities, are listed as below:

1. Eat more bread, especially wholemeal bread.

2. Eat more potatoes. Both bread and potatoes are excellent fillers, and need not be fattening if you don't load them with butter or fry them in fat.

3. Eat a high-fibre breakfast cereal but go easy on the sugar. The more bran a cereal contains, the higher is its fibre content.

4. Increase your intake of beans, peas, lentils and other pulses; consume meat sparingly.

5. Eat more vegetables. Vegetables, particularly the green leafy ones, are high in fibre. But don't overcook them or you will lose a lot of their goodness. Just cook enough to soften them.

6. Eat plenty of fresh fruits and salads. Even the softer fruits like melons or oranges contain fibre. Also, because fruits and vegetables contain a lot of water, they are low in calories and can help you stay slim.

7. Do not peel fruits and vegetables; leave the skin and eat it, e.g. you can eat whole baked or boiled potato with skin.

8. Sprinkle whole grain cereals on vegetable dishes before serving.

9. Make room for all the good food by cutting down on sugary and fatty items like biscuits, sweets and crisps especially between meals.

10. Try using wholemeal products.

11. Try brown rice. It takes longer to cook, but doesn't clump together into a sticky mess as white rice sometimes does.

21

Reduce Your Body Weight

*Facts are facts and will not disappear on account of
your likes.*

JAWAHAR LAL NEHRU

Before you know whether you are overweight or not, it is
essential to know your desirable body weight. The body
weight chart as developed by the Life Insurance Corporation
of India provides the desirable body weight for Indian men
and women (see p. 134)

Desirable Body Weight After Age 25: All health-conscious
people must have a good weighing machine in their homes.
Weigh yourself with light clothes (no coat or sweaters).
Remember that your weight fluctuates during the day. The
weight is usually more in the evening. It is best to weigh
yourself in the morning before breakfast. In any case, to find
out if you are gaining or losing weight, it is essential that you
weigh yourself under similar conditions on all occasions.

Is Obesity Hereditary? Questions have been raised for many
years regarding the role of heredity in causing obesity.
Although many people continue to believe that genes play
an important role in obesity, a recent study failed to find any
real evidence for genetics to take the blame. In the words of
Dr David Levitsky, professor of nutrition at Cornell University

Ideal Height/Weight Chart
Without Shoes

Height			Weight	
ft	in	cm	lbs	kg
Women over 25 years				
4	10	147.3	96 — 107	43.5 — 48.5
4	11	149.9	98 — 110	44.5 — 49.9
5	0	152.4	101 — 113	45.8 — 51.3
5	1	154.9	104 — 116	47.2 — 52.6
5	2	157.5	107 — 119	48.5 — 54.0
5	3	160.0	110 — 122	49.9 — 55.3
5	4	162.6	113 — 126	51.3 — 57.2
5	5	165.1	116 — 130	52.6 — 59.0
5	6	167.6	120 — 135	54.4 — 61.2
5	7	170.2	124 — 139	56.2 — 63.0
5	8	172.7	128 — 143	58.1 — 64.9
5	9	175.3	132 — 147	59.9 — 66.7
5	10	177.8	136 — 151	61.7 — 68.5
5	11	180.3	140 — 155	63.5 — 70.3
6	0	182.9	144 — 159	65.3 — 72.0
Men over 25 years				
5	2	157.5	118 — 129	53.5 — 58.5
5	3	160.0	121 — 133	54.9 — 60.3
5	4	162.6	124 — 136	56.2 — 61.7
5	5	165.1	127 — 139	57.6 — 63.0
5	6	167.6	130 — 143	59.0 — 64.9
5	7	170.2	134 — 147	60.8 — 66.7
5	8	172.7	138 — 152	62.6 — 68.9
5	9	175.3	142 — 156	64.4 — 70.8
5	10	177.8	146 — 160	66.2 — 72.6
5	11	180.3	150 — 165	68.0 — 74.8
6	0	182.9	154 — 170	69.9 — 77.1
6	1	185.4	158 — 175	71.7 — 79.4
6	2	188.0	162 — 180	73.5 — 81.6

Source: Life Insurance Corporation of India.

Medical School: 'You can tell your genes to get lost. You can successfully lose excessive body weight by reducing the total calories and fat in your diet. If fatty food, particularly, is reduced substantially, your body metabolism functions better and you can successfully lose weight.'

Twenty Ways to Lose Weight

If you are overweight, losing weight is essential to reduce your chances of heart disease. Many people can successfully manage to lose weight and yet, within a few weeks, they tend to regain the same weight. To maintain desirable body weight, you need to radically change your eating habits. A quick weight loss is often the result of excessive loss of body water and protein. The protein and water loss is not good since it will be replaced as quickly as you lose it. The following steps can help you to achieve a satisfactory and consistent weight loss.

1. Cut down the total calories in your daily diet. Unless you reduce your calories, you cannot expect to come close to your desirable body weight.

2. Start exercising. Exercise will help you burn the extra calories and fat that has already been stored in your body.

3. While you are reducing your caloric intake, ensure that you do take foods that are rich in vitamins and minerals.

4. Reduce the intake of fat and cholesterol as much as possible. Stay away from fried foods.

5. Most fat diets and diet pills do not work satisfactorily. Stay away from these gimmicks.

6. Maintain a record of what you eat. If you have failed to lose weight on last week's menu, make other necessary changes. Record keeping will help you to monitor your progress.

7. Stay away from snacks including chocolates and nuts.

8. Spend less time in the kitchen. The more time you spend in the kitchen, the more you are likely to eat.

9. Always go for smaller portions of food. Change your mental attitude towards food. Before you start eating, say to

yourself, 'I am only going to have a small portion. Even if the food is very tasty, I am determined not to overeat.'

10. Develop the habit of drinking a glass of water before your meals. The water will make you feel full in your stomach and, therefore, you are likely to eat less.

11. Avoid being a big eater at parties. Let no one put pressure on you to overeat. Excessive persuasion to eat more is considered to be a sign of hospitality, especially, in India.

12. Do not always try to finish everything on your plate. The extra calories, once deposited in your body as fat, are not easy to get rid of.

13. Avoid foods that contain too much sugar. One teaspoon of sugar has 16 calories. Some people take 10-20 teaspoonfuls of sugar in various drinks without realising the excessive calories they are taking.

14. Increase the amount of cereals, fruits and vegetables in your daily diet.

15. Remind yourself that you have been thinner in the past. Put out some photographs of a thinner 'you' and say to yourself, 'I have been like that, and I know that I can look like that again with my efforts.'

16. Do not start believing the myths about being overweight. A common myth in India is that you put on weight once you are married.

17. You do not have to accept being overweight with increasing age. Most people put on extra weight in their middle-age just because they are not exercising enough.

18. Remember that a man is recognized by the company he keeps. Avoid the company of people whose only pleasure in life is to keep eating. Keep at least two to three good friends who share your views against being overweight.

19. Monitor your progress and reward yourself for your success in losing weight.

20. When you do lose weight, change your clothes to your smaller size. Do not keep two sets of clothes just in case you regain your weight. Why give yourself a chance to put on that extra weight!

22

Make Exercising a Habit

True enjoyment comes from activity of the mind and exercise of the body; the two are ever united.
HUMBOLDT

Regular exercise is beneficial for your heart and your total health. There is no doubt that those who lead a physically active lifestyle are less likely to get heart disease as compared to those who have a lazy lifestyle. Many of those who have never been seriously interested in regular exercise may find it somewhat difficult to suddenly get into a routine of regular exercise. My usual suggestion to those who postpone exercising is to fix a definite date within the next two weeks and just start exercising! However, before you start any serious exercising programme, answer the following Medical History Questionnaire. If you answer 'yes' to any of these questions, no matter what your age is, it is mandatory that you visit a doctor before engaging in vigorous exercise, as overindulgence in exercise may put your heart under severe stress and strain.

On your visit to your doctor, discuss your plans, and have your blood pressure and heart examined. If your heartbeats are irregular, or if you are found to have a heart murmur or high blood pressure, you may not be ready to start exercising. So for your own safety, you do need a check-up.

If you answer 'Yes' to any question—Consult Your Doctor

	YES	NO
1. Has your doctor ever said you have heart trouble?	☐	☐
2. Do you frequently have pains in your chest?	☐	☐
3. Have you ever had an abnormal electrocardiogram (ECG) either while resting or exercising?	☐	☐
4. Have you ever had sensations of irregular or 'skipped' heart beats?	☐	☐
5. Do you often feel faint or have severe dizziness?	☐	☐
6. Do you have diabetes, high cholesterol, family history of heart disease, or smoke more than a pack and a half of cigarettes a day?	☐	☐
7. Has a doctor ever said that your blood pressure was too high?	☐	☐
8. Has a doctor ever told you that you have a bone or joint problem that has been aggravated by exercise?	☐	☐
9. Are you over the age of 60 and not accustomed to vigorous exercise?	☐	☐
10. Is there some other physical reason why you know you perhaps should not get into an active physical program even if you want to?	☐	☐

Types of Exercise

There are two main types of exercise: isotonic or aerobic; isometric or non-aerobic.

Aerobic Exercises are meant to increase the body's oxygen intake. They involve movement and the use of large muscle groups. Examples are walking, swimming, jogging

1. *Preventing Heart Disease: Exercising for a Healthy Heart*, Paul Vodak, Orient Paperbacks (1995); 45.

and running. Aerobic exercises raise your metabolic rate for several hours, so you continue to burn calories long after you have stopped exercising. These exercises are particularly recommended for cardiovascular benefits. Bicycling, skating and dancing are other forms of aerobic exercise.

Weight loss, better muscle tone and stamina are some of the main advantages of aerobic exercise. In terms of caloric loss for weight reduction, it may be worthwhile to know that in order to burn 100 calories, you could do one of the following exercises:

1. Walk 5 kilometres per hour for 25-30 minutes.
2. Walk 6 kilometres per hour for 23 minutes.
3. Walk 6.5 kilometres per hour for 17 minutes.
4. Run 1.5 kilometres for 10 minutes.
5. Do brisk walking for 20 minutes.
6. Go cycling at a moderate speed for 4 kilometres.
7. Climb stairs at a moderate pace for 10 minutes.
8. Walk on a treadmill 7 kilometres per hour, for 10 minutes.
9. Swim 1 kilometre per hour for 20-25 minutes.
10. Play badminton (singles)—for 20 minutes.

Non-aerobic Exercises are mainly used for body-building purposes. Muscle tensing is the underlying mechanism in isometric exercises. Good examples are press-ups or weightlifting. Isometric exercises result in the constriction of blood vessels, and this causes an increase in blood pressure. This type of exercise is not usually advised for people with high blood pressure or heart disease.

Benefits of Regular Exercise

The benefits and justification for regular exercise cannot be questioned. Based on scientific facts, regular exercise gives you the following benefits:

Weight Loss: Regular exercise means that you are burning extra calories on a daily basis. Unless you start overeating, you can expect a steady weight loss with regular exercise.

The total loss of weight will depend on the amount and the type of exercise. Millions of adults in their middle years tend to gain between 9-18 kg of extra body weight. With moderate exercise, a weight loss of 9-18 kg after 12-18 months is not unusual. Wouldn't it be nice to lose all that flab? Being overweight is a definite risk factor for heart disease. Weight reduction can reduce your risk of a heart attack.

Lowering of Blood Cholesterol: Regular physical exercise, especially the aerobic type, is known to result in an increased level of HDL and reduction in LDL. Although in most cases, exercise alone may result in only modest alteration, these beneficial changes are specially pronounced in obese adults who manage to lose between 5-15% of their body weight as a result of regular exercise and dietary changes. Several studies have noted that physically active persons tend to have higher HDL and lower LDL levels as compared to those with sedentary habits.

Although the precise mechanism remains unclear, the increase in HDL and reduction in LDL is thought to be caused by an increased metabolism of lipids, both during and after a period of physical exercise. This process is affected by an enhanced activity of a group of enzymes located at various receptor sites in the muscles and the fatty tissue. At least three different enzymes including lipoprotein lipase, lecithin-cholesterol-acyl-transferase (LCAT) and hepatic lipase are involved in this rather complex mechanism that leads to a favourable reduction in the LDL cholesterol and a rise in the HDL cholesterol.

Control of Blood Pressure: High blood pressure puts a strain on the walls of the blood vessels. Such blood vessels are more viable to collection of cholesterol within their walls, thus narrowing their lumen or inner cavity.

As seen above, exercise helps in the reduction of LDL which, in turn, lessens the availability of bad cholesterol and subsequent narrowing of arteries. Though the benefit of exercise in this case is an indirect one, its importance should not be undermined.

Prevention of Coronary Heart Disease: Heart muscle works better with regular exercise. The heart of an athlete can work more effectively and has a lower oxygen requirement. Regular exercise can stop the narrowing and hardening of your coronary arteries (atherosclerosis). Moreover, as a result of regular exercise, your heart develops extra blood channels that ensure a better and improved blood supply to the heart muscle, thereby helping to prevent the development of coronary heart disease.

Reduction in the Risk of Other Diseases:

Diabetes mellitus: Regular exercise reduces your risk of developing diabetes mellitus, especially the form of diabetes that is commonly seen in obese people after the age of 35 (type II diabetes).

Gallstones: Obese people have an increased chance of developing stones in their gall bladders. Those who exercise regularly are noted to have a lower rate of gallstones.

Stroke: Exercise reduces your risk of stroke by lowering your blood pressure and also reducing the hardening of the arteries of your brain.

Circulatory diseases: The incidence of peripheral vascular disease is lower in those individuals who participate in regular exercise programmes.

Improvement of General Well-being: Regular exercise helps in increasing your overall body resistance and endurance. The prevalence of anxiety and depression is much lower in those who exercise regularly as well.

Strengthening of Bones and Joints: Exercise strengthens your bones, joints, muscles and ligaments. Those who exercise remain fit and active till later years of life. Osteoporosis, a condition in which the bones become brittle and break easily, is less common in those who exercise regularly.

Improvement in Sexual Vigour: Exercise provides numerous other benefits. It has been noted that exercise can improve your sex life as well. Remember, sexual fitness goes with general body fitness.

Exercise and Heart Rate

There has been a lot of debate regarding the heart rate during exercise. A normal person has a resting heart (pulse) rate of between 70-75 beats per minute. After 1-2 months of regular exercise, you can expect to have a resting pulse rate of between 60-70 beats per minute. During the 20-30 minutes of your exercise time, your pulse rate rises. You should, however, not let your pulse go above 220, minus your age. For example, if you are 40 years old, do not let your pulse rate go above 220-40=180 beats per minute; this is your upper limit. Seventy per cent of 180 gives you a target heart rate of 126. What about your lower limit? If, during exercise, your pulse rate has gone from your resting pulse of 75 to only 85, perhaps you are not exercising vigorously enough. A range of 25 below the maximum rate, for example, for a 40-year-old, achieving a pulse rate of 155 to 180 beats per minute during exercise, would be considered desirable. Patients taking beta-blocking agents for hypertension or CHD normally have a lower pulse rate and, thus, their pulse rate may not increase very much during exercise. Elderly people also fail to show a substantial increase in their pulse rate during exercise.

Common Misconceptions about Exercise

Some of the common misconceptions about exercise that I have frequently encountered with Indian patients are reflected and addressed by the following questions and answers:

1. *Does exercise lead to an increase in appetite? Won't my weight go up if I exercise regularly?*

Exercise makes your body burn extra fat and calories. Exercise does not increase your appetite. In fact body weight reduction is best achieved through regular exercise and

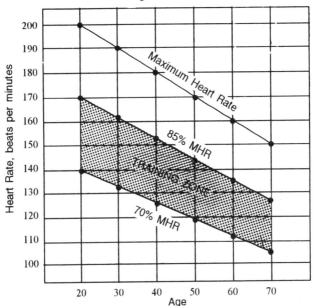

Maximum Heart Rate
and Training Heart Rate Zone

Estimated maximum heart rate and calculated training heart rates (70-85% MHR) for various ages. If actual MHR is known, calculate 70-85% of real value to determine training heart rate zone.

reduced calories intake. Those who just diet and neglect to exercise on a regular basis experience a loss of muscle tone and a feeling of weakness.

2. *If I remain busy doing different things in my office or at home, do I still need exercise?*

Keeping yourself active at the work place and home is good. However, physical exercise involves a coordinated action of your muscles, heart and body. Keeping busy with day-to-day chores is, of course, much better than leading a lazy lifestyle, but 20-30 minutes of sustained exercise has added advantages for your heart, lungs, brain and other organs.

2. *Preventing Heart Disease: Exercising for a Healthy Heart,* Paul Vodak, Orient Paperbacks (1995); 30.

3. *If I am tired and feel a lack of energy due to my daily work schedule, how can I really get involved with exercising?*

Regular exercise strengthens your muscles, heart and lungs. These vital organs will learn how to utilize oxygen more efficiently after you start doing exercise, making you feel stronger and more energetic. In fact, if you become easily tired, your muscles most likely need toning. The best way to accomplish this is to take regular exercise.

4. *Some people believe in the concept of No Pain, No Gain. Do I really need to continue exercising till my body starts aching?*

The best way to get the most out of exercising is to start slowly and keep exercising in moderation. Recent reports have confirmed that 20-30 minutes of daily exercise is all that you need. An excess of everything is bad and the same applies to exercise. Excessive exercising can cause muscle pain and fatigue.

5. *If I cannot exercise regularly, is it okay to do it on alternate days?*

Scientific studies have confirmed that for cardiovascular benefit, you need to do a minimum of 20-30 minutes exercise for, at least, 3 days a week. So, if for some reason, you cannot follow a 7-day schedule, an alternate-day-exercise programme is good enough.

Any good exercise programme must be followed in a regular fashion. If you stop for many weeks after just a few days of exercise, then exercise won't really improve your heart function. A lack of determination and commitment on your part is detrimental to the whole process. Though early morning exercise is well advised, the time during which you exercise may be adjusted according to your convenience or work schedule. For some, it may be easier to exercise in the evenings. Whatever the timings, ensure that you do not exercise soon after eating. Exercising should be an enjoyable activity; if done with a sense of boredom and tension, exercise is not likely to give you the expected positive results.

23

Coping with Stress

Anger and intolerance are the twin enemies of correct understanding.

MAHATMA GANDHI

With increasing industrialization and a faster pace of life, developing countries like India are also following the pattern set by Western nations. A stressful lifestyle resulting from day-to-day problems of finance, education, family and interpersonal relationships; as also the demands of work, travel, insecurity of job and business; and an urge to exceed and accomplish more than what you already possess—all lead to a degree of stress that results in slow but progressive damage to your cardiovascular system.

We tend to forget that the gradual damage to the coronary arteries (atherosclerosis) starts when we are in our early 20s, and by continuing with a stressful lifestyle, we are only enhancing the damage. A heart attack that occurs today, in fact, may have started very slowly many years ago with the gradual narrowing and hardening of the coronary arteries.

Are You Under Stress?

Stress is a time bomb that must be diffused. Answer the following questionnaire to find out if you are under stress. Answer YES or NO for each question.

Check Your Stress Level

	Yes	No
1. Have you been committing an increasing number of mistakes at work?	☐	☐
2. Have you been suffering from frequent colds and infections?	☐	☐
3. Have you been getting frequent tension headaches?	☐	☐
4. Are you getting aches and pains all over your body regularly?	☐	☐
5. Have you been getting frequent short periods of restlessness and anxiety?	☐	☐
6. Do you always feel tired and a lack of energy?	☐	☐
7. Has your sleep pattern changed recently? Do you experience difficulty in sleeping or wake up several times during the night?	☐	☐
8. Are you experiencing periods of palpitation? (missed or irregular heartbeat)	☐	☐
9. Have you been getting frequent episodes of heartburn?	☐	☐
10. Have you been increasing your intake of alcohol lately?	☐	☐
11. Have you increased your smoking lately?	☐	☐
12. Have you been feeling depressed lately?	☐	☐
13. Have you been noted to indulge in nail biting?	☐	☐
14. Have you been taking tranquillizers to calm your nerves?	☐	☐
15. Have you been getting into excessive arguments with your colleagues or family members?	☐	☐
16. Is your blood pressure higher than usual?	☐	☐
17. Has your appetite diminished lately?	☐	☐
18. Have you lost weight even though you did not plan to do so?	☐	☐
19. Have you lost interest in your hobbies?	☐	☐
20. Do you generally feel that you are lacking fun in your life?	☐	☐

Interpret Your Responses

Count the number of 'Yes' responses. If your total number of 'Yes' responses is between 0-4, you have low stress; 4-8 means a medium degree of stress; a score of over 8 is indicative of a high degree of stress. Clearly the more the 'Yes' responses, the higher is your stress level.

How to Reduce Stress

❑ Do not get upset over minor matters. You will often hear people saying: 'If something goes wrong, I just cannot stand it. That is the way I am.' Some of these people seem to enjoy an air of superiority while saying so. The fact is that getting upset is simply against the stability of your biochemical equilibrium. Anger and frustration are associated with the secretion of a number of hormones that can increase your cholesterol and also raise your blood pressure. You may really be wasting a lot of your valuable and enjoyable time by getting upset over trivial matters.

❑ Create a joyful environment for yourself. Some people wrongly assume that joyful living is only for young children and a mature person should, somehow, not appear to be joyful. Why not do things that really bring pleasure to your life?

❑ Find new hobbies and interests. Do something different. People who have a fixed and rigid life day after day can easily become bored. A dull lifestyle is a recipe for excessive stress.

❑ Have, at least, a few friends of jovial nature who can create an environment of fun, pleasure and enthusiasm. A person with a persistently pessimistic attitude cannot be expected to bring fun and excitement into your life.

❑ Develop the habit of smiling and laughing. Laughter, in fact, is the best medicine for stress and stress-related diseases. Smiling and laughing can bring about positive changes in your body hormones. Reducing your stress level can, not only protect you from heart disease, but also enhance your quality of life enormously.

24

Say 'No' to Smoking

It does not take much strength to do things, but it requires great strength to decide on what to do.

ELBERT HUBBARD

During the last thirty years, millions of people in countries like the United States and England have realized the dangers of smoking and stopped smoking. During the same period, millions of Indians have picked up smoking habits. It has been noted that if the older members of the family including parents, grandparents, uncles, and even older brothers and cousins are smokers, it does not take long for the younger members of the family to pick up these bad habits and start smoking. Many children grow up with the notion that smoking is just a normal part of life. It may be years before they realize that smoking is harmful for their health. For many, it is too late, since they have now become very addicted to the nicotine in the tobacco!

Smoking increases your risk of heart attack. An average smoker is, at least, twice at risk of a sudden heart attack. Nicotine causes narrowing of the coronary arteries and promotes the clumping of blood cells—the platelets. A 25-year-old man smoking two packs of cigarettes a day, is expected to die, at least, eight years before a non-smoking person of the same age. Stameler and Epstein studied the relationship of smoking with heart attacks and deaths. They observed men between the ages of 30-59 years for a period of ten years and found that non-smokers had a 40/1,000 death ratio due to heart attacks. Adults smoking half a pack of cigarettes per day had 66/1,000 death ratio due to heart attacks. Adults smoking more than one pack of cigarettes per day had a 131/1,000 death ratio due to heart attacks.

Steps to Stop Smoking

1. Plan a definite date for quitting smoking within the next seven to ten days. Do not leave the decision for months.

2. Remind yourself about the dangers of smoking. In particular, think of the disasters of a sudden heart attack, cancer or stroke.

3. Remind yourself that smoking can shorten your life by several years. Ask yourself repeatedly: 'Do I need to kill myself at a premature age because of my continued smoking?'

4. If you have failed in your efforts to stop smoking in the past, do not be discouraged. There are many who have succeeded at quitting smoking with firm determination and will-power. It may take 4-10 attempts to quit smoking forever.

5. Think of the amount of money you are losing because of your continued smoking.

6. Create a recording system for yourself. Maintain a diary and record your success and failures.

7. Do not offer or accept a cigarette from anyone.

8. In the initial days after you stop smoking, you may get an occasional urge to smoke. Plan to direct your attention to something else during these episodes of increased urge. For example, take chewing gum, or have a banana or an apple instead of smoking a cigarette.

9. Nicotine chewing-gums are available in some countries and have been used for dealing with the withdrawal effect of nicotine addiction such as irritability, lack of concentration, depression, headaches and lethargy. If you are experiencing one or more of these symptoms, then you must see your doctor.

149

10. Do not be afraid of gaining a few kilograms in weight when quitting smoking. Less than 50% smokers tend to gain some weight. Remember, you will have to gain 23-45 kg in weight to approximate the health risk of continued smoking. Do not let yourself continue smoking just because you are scared of gaining a few kilograms of weight. With an active lifestyle and dietary restrictions, the weight gain should not become a problem.

The simple fact is that smoking has no virtues and, therefore, there is simply no justification for you to continue smoking. You owe it to yourself to stop smoking now!

25

Moderate Your Alcohol Consumption

Ninety-nine per cent of the failures come from people who have the habit of making excuses.
GEORGE W. CARVER

Alcohol abuse is a common problem. Many people have a problem accepting the fact that they drink excessively. Some who take six to eight drinks per day may only admit to two or three drinks per day. I am reminded of my earlier years in medical training when I was told by a senior consultant in England to multiply the number of drinks by at least two if I wanted an accurate estimate of the alcohol consumption in a suspected alcoholic.

Family members and close friends are almost always good at recognizing the problem of excessive alcohol abuse. If you or your family members have any doubt about alcohol abuse, a simple test called the Michigan Alcoholism Screening Test (MAST questionnaire) can help you to confirm your suspicion of alcoholism. Answer the following questions in either. YES or No and then examine your responses. Do you have more YES responses than you expected? You may be surprised. Even 2 or 3 YES responses may be suggestive of alcoholism.

Mast Questionnaire (Modified Version)

	Yes	No
1. Do you feel you are a normal drinker and drink less than three times a month?	☐	☐
2. Have you ever awakened in the morning and found that you couldn't remember a part of the evening because you were drinking?	☐	☐
3. Does your spouse, a parent or other close relative ever worry or complain about your drinking?	☐	☐
4. Can you stop drinking without a struggle after one or two drinks? Do you ever feel guilty about your drinking?	☐	☐
5. Have you been involved in a physical fight during or soon after drinking?	☐	☐
6. Has drinking ever created problems between you and your spouse, family members or close friends?	☐	☐
7. Have you run into problems at work because of your drinking?	☐	☐
8. Have you ever lost a job because of drinking?	☐	☐
9. Have you ever neglected your obligations, your work or other commitments for two or more days in a row because of drinking?	☐	☐
10. Do you drink before noon fairly often?	☐	☐
11. Have you ever been told that you have liver trouble or cirrhosis?	☐	☐
12. After heavy drinking, have you ever had severe shaking or delirium tremens (DTs), or heard voices, or seen things that were not really there?	☐	☐
13. Have you ever gone to anyone for help about your drinking?	☐	☐

14. Have you ever been in a hospital ☐ ☐
    (medical or psychiatric) because of
    your drinking?
15. Have you ever had legal problems ☐ ☐
    because of your alcoholic abuse
    (driving under the influence of alcohol)?

Unfortunately there is an increasing trend towards alcohol use in India today. We drink when a child is born; many drink to mourn a death in the family. Festivals like Diwali, Holi, Christmas and New Year are big occasions for people to drink. Marriage receptions are now considered almost incomplete if there are no arrangements for drinks. Guests and close friends often get offended if they are not served their favourable drinks at these functions. Transfers and promotions have become common excuses for big cocktail parties. Unfortunately, someone who does not drink at all—a teetotaller—is often considered a 'backward' person. Is it very difficult then to see why we have an increasing emphasis on drinking alchohol in our society today?

A social drinker is someone who drinks only on social occasions such as birthdays and marriages, probably, not more than ten to twenty times per year. You suffer from alcoholism only if you have become addicted to alcohol. Alcoholism, in fact, is a chronic and progressive medical disease that usually develops over a period of five to ten years. Alcoholism commonly leads to alcohol dependence, health, social and even legal problems. Alcoholics cannot function properly without alcohol; withdrawal of alcohol may cause delirium tremens and convulsions.

Alcohol abuse can lead to several medical problems. Your liver, heart, brain, kidneys, nerves and muscles may all be damaged by prolonged and excessive alcohol intake. It is estimated that regular intake of more that 60 ml of alcohol in men and 40 ml of alcohol per day in women can cause serious problems after 5-7 years.

Corrective Measures

There are several ways in which you can help yourself to reduce and even stop your drinking.

Self-help: 'God helps those who help themselves' is a well-known saying. If you strongly believe that you want to free yourself from the clutches of alcohol dependency, surely you can do a lot for yourself. Strong determination and will-power can help you achieve the right results. As a first step, you must reduce the number of drinks per week slowly. For example, if you have been taking five drinks per day, reduce your quota to four drinks per day. Give yourself at least three to four weeks before you make another reduction. Remember, if your body cells have become addicted to alcohol over a period of many years, it will certainly require many weeks to bring the body cells back to their independent living without alcohol. Once you feel confident and you can manage two to three drinks per day as compared to your previous level of five to six drinks, you are ready to take a complete break from alcohol for one to two days per week. Withdrawal symptoms can be severe in someone who has been drinking heavily for many years. Close supervision and help from your doctor is necessary. While you are reducing your alcohol intake, start doing regular exercises. Good quality nutrition with high protein and vitamins is essential. Yoga and meditation can also help you keep your nerves under control.

Seek Help from Your Family and Friends: The spouse and all grown-up children must participate actively in helping an alcoholic person. It is important that the family members and close friends do not encourage drinking during socialization. Joining a group of friends who are almost in the same age group and are also keen to reduce or stop drinking can be very beneficial. By meeting frequently, you can share your fear, loneliness, anger and anxiety about your current situation. Do not be afraid of your failures.

Take Your Doctor's Advice: Seeking help from your doctor is essential. Your physician can discuss your alcohol-related problems and point out if any of your organs have been affected by alcohol abuse. In addition to your regular physician, you may also need the help of a psychiatrist who is, usually, better trained to understand the emotional and psychological aspect of drinking. Unfortunately, many people in India tend to think wrongly that only crazy people need to go to psychiatrists. Just as a good physician can cure your physical health, a good psychiatrist can do a lot to cure your mental health. A desire to drink excessively results both from physical as well as psychological dependence on alcohol. Your doctor may also decide to prescribe Antabuse (disulfiram) therapy for your drinking. Antabuse is a drug that interferes with the metabolism of alcohol in your liver and produces a chemical in your blood. Upon drinking alcohol, a person on Antabuse treatment experiences severe headache, flushing, nausea and vomiting. This kind of a 'shocking' experience makes the alcoholic stay away from alcohol.

Contact Alcoholic Anonymous (AA): The services of AA are available in over 100 countries, including India. AA is a voluntary organization that started many years ago in the United States. The philosophy of AA is to help the individual through advice, encouragement and counselling. AA can also put you in touch with many others who have successfully stopped drinking. AA is certainly not a replacement for your doctor or family. This organization can provide you with much needed friendship, warmth, support and guidance that can prove to be very helpful in your success against alcoholism.

In conclusion, excessive drinking is dangerous for your body. There is little doubt that alcoholism can shorten your lifespan by several years. With a strong will-power, determination and consistent efforts, there is no reason why you cannot stop drinking now!

26

The Role of Vitamins and Antioxidants

Medicines are nothing in themselves, if not properly used, but the very hands of the Gods, if employed with reason and prudence.

HEROPHILUS

Multiple chemical reactions continue to occur in your body cells at all times including your sleeping hours. As a result of these metabolic reactions, certain unstable particles or toxins are produced in the body cells. These toxins are often called free radicals. It is believed that these free radicals slowly damage your body cells and cause aging, degeneration of the cells and even cancers of various types.

In recent years, it has been suggested that free radicals may even be contributing towards a heart attack. Researchers from Texas and California have reported that cholesterol exists and circulates in the blood. This can be converted into a harmful form of cholesterol by the free radicals, thereby leading to the clogging of the arteries and causing atherosclerosis, and, possibly, a heart attack.

Beta-Carotene, Vitamins C and E

Latest studies reveal that beta-carotene and vitamins C and E are antioxidants or agents which reduce oxidation and successfully counter the damaging effects of the free radicals.

A major recent study reported that high intake of

antioxidants like beta-carotene can significantly reduce the rate of heart disease. Dr Charles Hennekens from the well-known Brigham and Women's Hospital in Boston presented some interesting results from the Physician's Health Study, a 10-year project involving 22,000 male doctors who are being studied in detail to find out if the intake of beta-carotene, aspirin, or both would really influence the rate of heart disease. From a small group of 333 men, early results have indicated that men taking beta-carotene supplements get 40% fewer heart attacks than those not taking any additional beta-carotene. The study itself is still continuing and more information will be made available within a period of 2 to 3 years at the conclusion of the full study. Those getting fewer heart attacks in the study were being given 50 mg of carotene per day, which is approximately two cups of cooked carrots. It has been suggested that at least 25 mg of carotene is required per day to cut down your risk of heart disease. Most people, unfortunately, take only 1.5-2 mg per day.

Other similar studies have also found convincing evidence that increased beta-carotene intake can reduce the risk of heart attack. In a study conducted at Johns Hopkins University Medical School, researchers found that there was a 50% reduction in the rate of heart attack in a group of people taking large amounts of beta-carotene. Dr R.A. Riemersma and his colleagues from the University of Edinburgh collaborated with some researchers from the University of Berne in Switzerland and conducted a study. The idea of this project was to find out if the blood concentration of antioxidant vitamins such as carotene and vitamins C and E influenced the risk of angina or not. Three hundred and ninety-four healthy persons were compared with 110 patients suffering from angina. Multiple health questions as contained in the World Health Organization Chest Pain Questionnaire were answered by all participants. In addition, blood samples were tested to find out the blood level of antioxidants. Patients with angina were often heavy smokers and it was clear from blood results that angina patients who smoked had a lower concentration of carotene, and vitamins C and E in their blood. Even in the healthy 394 people, smokers had lower levels of these vitamins. The ex-smokers, interestingly, were found to have better vitamin C and carotene levels than those who were still smoking. It was concluded that smokers with heart disease had a much lower concentration of these antioxidants. The researchers even stated: 'Because food processing often destroys natural antioxidants, and because some people tend to take in little quantities of vitamins C and E, populations with a high incidence of heart disease should supplement their eating habits with more cereals, fruits and vegetables, and vitamin E-rich products'.

Besides controlling the increase of oxidized LDL cholesterol that can cause clogging of the arteries, there may be other ways that the antioxidants may help. Results from the Baltimore Longitudinal Study on aging, conducted by the National Institute of Aging, confirmed that people with high blood levels of vitamin C tend to have a high concentration of HDL, the good cholesterol that reduces the risk of heart attack. Studies from Tufts University have, similarly, reported that people with high vitamin C blood levels more commonly have normal blood pressures as compared to those with low vitamin C levels. We know for sure that high blood pressure increases the risk of heart disease. It is quite possible that vitamin C, by keeping the blood pressure within normal range, reduces the risk of heart disease.

Thus we see that antioxidant nutrients may help protect you from heart disease. The metabolic toxins or the free radicals that accumulate in your body are thought to play an important role, not only in the aging process and cancer, but also in the initiation of the process of atherosclerosis. All this starts with the oxidization of the LDL cholesterol which

Good Sources of Beta-Carotene, Vitamin C and Vitamin E

Beta-carotene	Vitamin C	Vitamin E
Apricots	Citrus fruits & juices (orange & lemon)	Wheat germ
Carrots	Tomato & tomato Juice	Soyabean
Mangoes	Cabbage	Wholegrain cereals
Papayas	Potatoes	Corn
Pumpkin	Green peppers	Nuts
Spinach	(capsicum)	Seeds
Sweet potatoes	Mangoes	Peppers
Turnips	Guavas	Carrots
Coriander leaves	Strawberries	Green leafy vegetables
Peaches		

gets deposited in the walls of your arteries. Antioxidants can stop the oxidation of LDL and, therefore, save you from atherosclerosis. With the intake of a higher amount of foods containing beta-carotene, vitamins C and E, you will have a greater opportunity to reduce your risk of heart disease.

27

Prescription Drugs for Cholesterol Treatment

*Poison and medicine are often the same substance
given with different intents.*

PETER MERE LATHAM

The first step in the war against high cholesterol is to make the necessary changes in your diet. Dietary changes are completely safe and, fortunately, many people do not require anything more than a simple diet change to bring their cholesterol back to normal levels.

The treatment of high cholesterol is a lifelong commitment. I am sure that if you can control your cholesterol only by making changes in the diet, you would be happy to avoid taking tablets. Besides inconvenience, the side-effects and the cost are two major problems associated with taking tablets. Most patients on cholesterol-lowering drug treatment require frequent blood tests to find out if their liver is still functioning well or not.

Dietary changes must first be discussed thoroughly with your doctor before being undertaken. If the changes in the diet do not help, your physician can suggest further dietary modifications. Some people give up too easily on dietary changes as they fail to take to a low cholesterol and low fat diet. If you are aware that you are cheating yourself with in-between snacks, chocolates, and so on, it may be wise to

160

start once again with dietary changes. You must give yourself enough time—at least 6-9 months—with strict dietary control before you start taking medication to lower the cholesterol. It is estimated that up to 85 per cent of adults can successfully lower their cholesterol with diet alone. The remaining 15% per cent will need to take tablets along with dietary control. If dietary changes fail to control high cholesterol, then, in addition to dietary changes, drugs are recommended. The goal of the treatment is to reduce the total cholesterol to below 200 mg, and LDL to below 130 mg.

Commonly Used Drugs

The following are some of the commonly used medications for lowering cholesterol (trade names vary in different countries):

- Bile acid sequestrants
- Nicotinic acid *(niacin)*
- Fibric acids *(clofibrate, gemfibrozil)*
- HMF CoA reductase inhibitors
- *Probucol*

Different medications have different modes of action. Though in most patients, one type of medication alone may be enough to control high cholesterol, in special circumstances, your physician may prefer to prescribe more than one type of medication.

Bile Acid Sequestrants: Drugs from the bile acid sequestrants group include *cholestyramine* (trade name—QUESTRAN) and *colestripol* (trade name—COLESTID). These drugs bind bile acids in the intestine—the digestive tube. The bile acid is constantly being formed by the liver and is released in the intestine where it is required mainly for the digestion and absorption of fat. From the intestine, a large part of the bile acid is reabsorbed by the liver. Bile acid sequestrants bind the bile acids and thus interfere with its absorption. A lot of cholesterol is required for the formation of bile acids. With the elimination of the bile acids, the cholesterol level declines.

161

The Lipid Research Clinic Coronary Primary Prevention trial, that involved nearly 4,000 patients, used *cholestyramine* and found that the total cholesterol dropped by 13%; LDL was reduced by 20-35%, depending upon the amount of drug used. It has been noted that, usually, cholesterol is lowered within 3-4 weeks after starting the treatment. In most cases, an LDL reduction of 15-25% can be expected. Common side-effects of bile acid binding drugs include constipation, nausea and flatulence. *Cholestyramine* is usually taken in an 8 gm dose twice a day, that is, a total of 16 gm per day. It is important to start with a lower dose and slowly increase the dose. Not all patients require a full dose of 16 gm per day. Constipation can be relieved by taking a high fibre diet or even a laxative. If you are taking some other medications for your heart condition such as beta-blockers, digoxin or warfarin, then bile acid binding drugs may sometime interfere with their absorption. It is helpful if you take these drugs 1-2 hours before taking *cholestyramine*. Although the bile acid binding drugs are good for reducing total and LDL cholesterol, your blood triglycerides may be increased. All cholesterol-lowering drugs must be taken only with the guidance and supervision of your doctor.

Nicotinic Acid (Niacin): Nicotinic acid interferes with the synthesis of VLDL lipoproteins, a form of bad cholesterol, in the liver. The total cholesterol and the LDL levels decline and the HDL levels are increased. In scientific studies, nicotinic acid has been found to reduce the rate of second heart attacks and death in heart disease patients.

A dose of 3-6 gm per day is usually necessary to produce a significant decrease of cholesterol. It is best to start with smaller doses of 50 mg, 2-3 times per day, and then increase slowly over a period of several weeks. Since larger doses can cause serious side-effects, niacin must be taken only under the supervision of your doctor. Side-effects include flushing, itching, gastric pain, nausea and vomiting. Niacin is best if taken after meals. Taking one aspirin tablet thirty minutes before Niacin can also help prevent the problem of flushing. Niacin can also increase your blood sugar. So if you happen to be a diabetic, it is all the more important that you do not take niacin without first consulting your doctor.

Fibric Acids: The two most commonly used fibric acids are *gemfibrozil* (LOPID) and *clofibrate* (ATROMID). Fibric acids have a rather complex mechanism of action in cholesterol synthesis and disposal. The net effect is to lower the total and LDL cholesterol and triglycerides. There is a beneficial rise in the HDL as well. The total reduction of cholesterol and LDL is between 10-20% each. Clinical studies have established the role of fibric acids beyond any doubt. Side-effects include nausea and vomiting, muscle aches and pains, skin rashes, abnormal liver function and excessive gallstone formation. In some patients, the blood sugar may also rise. Once again, like other medications, fibric acid should be taken only under the guidance of your physician.

HMG CoA Reductase: Hydroxymethyl Glutaryl-coenzyme A Reductase is a recent group of medications that have really revolutionized the drug treatment of high cholesterol during the past five years. HMG A is an enzyme that is required in the liver for cholesterol formation. By interfering with the action of the enzyme, the drug stops the formation of cholesterol. *Lovastatin* (trade name—MEVACOR) is one of the many drugs that are being widely used to control high cholesterol today. The benefits are seen in the form of a low total and LDL cholesterol and triglycerides, and elevation of HDL cholesterol.

Although *lovastatin* is comparatively safe, side-effects do exist and these include liver cell dysfunction, muscle weakness and skin rashes. Periodic blood tests to check the liver functions are important. Some patients may even develop cataracts in their eyes and, therefore, regular eye check-ups are also recommended if you are taking this type of medication.

Probucol: Though the exact mechanism of this drug remains unclear, it reduces both total and LDL cholesterol. Unfortunately, because probucol also reduces the HDL cholesterol, the drug has not been widely used so far. The usual doses are 500 mg twice a day. Side-effects include nausea and vomiting, flatulence and heart beat irregularities. There is some suggestion that probucol may decrease the deposition of fat and cholesterol in the walls of the arteries but this requires further confirmation and more studies.

Are Two Drugs Better Than One?

The commonly accepted principle of treatment of any disease is that treatment with one drug is always better than using two drugs. However, the potential effect of two medications is such, that for quicker and more effective results, physicians may prefer to prescribe two drugs together. Since each type of cholesterol-lowering drug has a different mechanism of action, a combination of two drugs will prove to be more effective. If the maximum dose of one drug alone has failed to lower your cholesterol, you will, perhaps, need to take two drugs. Some patients simply cannot tolerate the maximum allowed dose of a particular drug and if so, will need to be treated with smaller doses of two cholesterol-lowering medications. Some commonly used combinations of drugs include the following:

Bile acid binding agents and nicotinic acids. This combination is used especially if the nicotinic acid alone is causing severe side-effects.

Bile acid binding agents and lovastatin. Satisfactory reduction in total and LDL cholesterol can be achieved with this combination of drugs without significant side-effects. Between 30-50% of the usual doses can be used and, therefore, the side-effects can be minimized.

Fibric acids and nicotinic acids. This combination is best suited for you if you have high total cholesterol, LDL and triglycerides. Bile acid binding agents are not effective in reducing the triglyceride levels.

164

The first step in winning the war against high cholesterol is to try to modify your diet for, at least, 6-9 months. Around 10-15% of adults with high cholesterol need to take drugs in addition to dietary changes. During the past ten years, we have acquired a better understanding of the use of cholesterol-lowering medications. Safer drugs have been developed. Some new agents are still being made available. All of this sounds very exciting and promising. However, the fact remains that drug treatment is not completely free from side-effects. All drugs, including cholesterol-lowering agents, should be taken only under the supervision and guidance of your own physician.

Fortunately, with the availability of a number of drugs, it has become much easier to control high cholesterol and reduce the risk of heart disease for millions of people today.

PART IV
A Healthy Future Is Yours

28

Heart Disease Can Be Reversed

*It is hard to fail, but it is worse never to have tried
to succeed. In this life we get nothing save by effort.*

THEODORE ROOSEVELT

By now you should have no doubt in your mind as to
whether high cholesterol is strongly associated with a
high risk of heart disease. More than 10 major scientific
studies have confirmed the relationship of high cholesterol
with increasing incidences of heart attacks and death.
Population studies from different countries have established
that if the average cholesterol of the population is high, the
people will suffer more heart attacks.

Until a few years ago many authorities doubted whether
the blockage in the coronary arteries could be reversed. During
the past ten years, however, several scientists have reported
that a reduction of cholesterol can make a significant
difference in the process of atherosclerosis—the clogging of
the arteries.

Low Fat Vegetarian Diet: A vegetarian diet comprising
steamed or boiled vegetables has a low fat content. However,
any extra fat, butter or *ghee* added, or deep frying of
vegetables, takes away the low fat quality of the vegetables.
If a cooking medium must be used, cooking oils containing

unsaturated fats should be preferred (see Chapter 16). One of the earliest studies relating to a low fat vegetarian diet was conducted in 1977 by Dr Antonio M. Gotto, Jr., Chief of Medicine at Baylor School of Medicine,Texas. A group of patients who had definite coronary heart disease confirmed by angiography, were put on a vegetarian diet, asked to do moderate exercise and undertake a stress management programme. After 30 days, several patients reported a significant reduction in the frequency and severity of angina, and their blood pressure was noted to have come down to a near-normal level. Exercise testing revealed that many of these patients could exercise an average of 50% more as a result of this 30-day treatment. In 1980, Dr Gotto repeated a similar study using more modern techniques to assess the change in the heart function as a result of dietary and lifestyle changes. Once again, the results were impressive with a more than 20% reduction in blood cholesterol and a mean 91% reduction in angina pains.

Drs Robert Wissler and Vesslinovitch have, through some pioneering experiments on monkeys, demonstrated the effectiveness of cholesterol lowering on the reversibility of the process of atherosclerosis in the arteries of monkeys. Medically speaking, monkeys closely resemble human beings. The results indicated that the hardening of the arteries or atherosclerosis can be induced in a period of 9-14 months in these monkeys if they are fed on a high fat, high cholesterol diet. Conversely, if given a low fat and low cholesterol diet, significant regression can be seen in the cholesterol deposition in the arteries of the monkeys.

Cholesterol-lowering Medication: A major study called Familial Atherosclerosis Treatment Study (FATS) confirmed that if the cholesterol is significantly lowered through diet and/or drugs, it would not only stop the progression of coronary heart disease, but would also lead to a decline in the fat that has already been deposited in the wall of the arteries. In other words, dissolving the fatty deposits from the walls of the arteries has been proved to be possible. The study involved 146 adults all below the age of sixty-two. Dr B. Greg Brown, from the University of Washington, thoroughly studied these patients. Apart from a clinical examination, all patients underwent a special examination of their coronary arteries through X-ray techniques (coronary angiography). The findings of the X-rays were analysed by special computer methods. It was noted that the patients who were not given any special treatment to lower their cholesterol showed an increase in the narrowing of their coronary arteries. Those who received drug treatment to lower the cholesterol showed a reduction in the narrowing of the coronary arteries. Patients who had a reversal of the narrowing of coronary arteries had a 75% reduction in the incidence of heart attacks and deaths as compared to those who showed an increase in narrowing of coronary arteries because of persistently high cholesterol levels. In an interview, Dr Brown commented that, initially, he was somewhat sceptical about the importance of aggressively lowering the cholesterol in patients with established coronary heart disease, but as a result of this study, he was convinced that cholesterol reduction could do wonders in reversing the process of atherosclerosis and reduction of heart disease.

The unblockage of the clogged coronary arteries has also been shown by Dr David Blankenhorn, Director of the University of Southern California Atherosclerosis Research Unit. Dr Blankenhorn's report in 1987 was the result of a two-and-a-half-year study of 162 men who had already undergone coronary artery bypass surgery. One group of patients was put on dietary changes and the other group was treated with diet and cholesterol-lowering medication (*niacin* and *cholestyramine*). This trial was called the cholesterol-lowering atherosclerosis study (CLAS). As many as 61% of the patients actively treated for lowering cholesterol demonstrated regression of atherosclerosis. Altogether, the results in those showing cholesterol reduction because of diet changes and use of cholesterol-lowering medications were highly suggestive of the regression of atherosclerosis.

Lifestyle Changes: In the summer of 1990, Dr Dean Ornish of the Preventive Medicine Research Institute in California published the beneficial results of cholesterol lowering in the *Lancet*, the world-renowned British medical journal. It was clearly shown that people with blocked coronary arteries can expect to unblock their arteries with positive changes in their lifestyle, which should include a strict vegetarian diet, stress reduction and regular exercises. Dr Clude Lenfant, Director of the National Heart, Lung and Blood Institute in Bethesda, United States, commented after this report that this study showed strong evidence that lifestyle changes alone can actually reduce the progression of coronary heart disease.

Let me give you some details of what Dr Ornish did to prove the effect of lifestyle changes on cholesterol and heart disease. Forty-one patients, 35-75 years old, were selected from different socio-economic and ethnic backgrounds. All of them had a definite diagnosis of coronary heart disease. Special X-ray techniques (coronary angiograms) had confirmed the presence of narrowing of coronary arteries in all patients. These 41 patients were then divided into two groups. One group of 22 patients were put on a programme of dietary changes (very low cholesterol and fat diet); daily exercises (walking half an hour per day); and stress reduction through breathing exercises, yoga and meditation. The remaining 19 patients were treated as standard American patients with few changes in their lifestyle or stress level. After one year, the X-ray pictures of the coronary arteries were repeated in all patients. Out of the 22 patients who followed lifestlye and dietary changes, 18 patients showed a remarkable unblocking of the coronary arteries: 3 showed minor unblocking of the arteries; one patient who failed to follow the programme showed progression of the narrowing of coronary arteries. What about the symptoms of heart disease? Most patients reported a major reduction in the frequency of chest pain. Out of the nineteen patients treated with the standard American approach, 10 showed progression of the blockage of coronary arteries. As a group, all these 19 patients reported a 165% rise in the frequency of chest pain, 95% rise in the duration, and a 39% rise in the severity of chest pain. A remarkable difference indeed!

As a result of several studies conducted so far, we now have clear evidence that a large reduction in blood cholesterol can definitely stop the further blockage of coronary arteries. In many cases, the arteries that have been blocked can open up. However, this does not mean complete elimination of fat and cholesterol from your diet. Dr Joseph Alpert from the University of Boston in the United States, points out that regression does not mean a complete 'no' to the use of fat in your diet. Switching from saturated to unsaturated fats can have a significant effect. It is estimated that a persistent cholesterol level of between 150-170 mg is required to unblock the coronary arteries. Merely bringing down the cholesterol to a 190-200 mg range may not be enough. In any case, the news about reversing the blockage of coronary arteries by lowering the cholesterol is very encouraging, and even if you have not been very careful in the past, you can still do a lot to benefit your coronary arteries now!

29

Treating Clogged Arteries: Surgical Methods

Surgery does the ideal thing--it separates the patient from his disease. It puts the patient back to bed and the disease in a bottle.

LOGAN CLENDENING

Medical treatment of coronary heart disease involves the use of drugs (digoxin, beta-blockers or calcium channel blockers) to maintain the force and regularity of contraction of the heart. Whenever possible, increasing the blood flow in the coronary arteries through the use of vasodilators has also been practised for many years. Unfortunately, it is not always possible to maintain adequate blood supply to the heart muscle through the use of medications. In such cases surgical procedures become necessary. Bypass heart surgery is perhaps the best-known procedure for heart disease patients.

Bypass Heart Surgery

Coronary artery bypass surgery has become a well-established way of treating selective patients over the past twenty years. More than 500,000 bypass operations are done each year around the world. Out of these, 250,000 are carried out in the United States alone. If you have coronary heart disease that cannot be effectively controlled with medication, or if you are noted to have a severe degree of disease in the left main coronary artery, or all the three branches, you probably need a bypass operation.

The procedure itself has become much safer in the hands of experienced surgeons in recent years. Since the first bypass surgery in the late 1960s, the average age of the bypass surgery patient has gone up by fifteen years. Today you can see thousands of patients over the age of sixty who are leading a good-quality life after a heart operation. In one study involving nearly 9,000 patients in the United States between 1975-1978, the death rate with this operation was noted to be 2.5%; over 90% of patients were found to live for five or more years after the surgery. Today the death rate due to bypass surgery in good American medical centres is less than 1%. In other words, more than 99% patients come out alive and well after the surgery.

Bypass surgery is now available in several medical centres in India. Most major cities including Bombay, Delhi, Calcutta and Madras have excellent facilities for bypass surgery. I am often asked if I could give a comparison between the heart surgery results of the Indian hospitals and the British or American hospitals. In the absence of published results, it is very difficult to compare the East with the West. The expenses are, of course, much higher when you have heart surgery in Western countries. On the question of comparison, one of my medical friends recently summarized it this way: Surgery is team work. Because of better operative and post-operative facilities, perhaps I would go and have the bypass at the best medical centre in the United States if I could afford it. If I cannot afford going abroad, then I am lucky to have the bypass available in India at a much lower cost'.

Bypass surgery is carried out on one or more coronary arteries. The idea of the operation is to stitch a new blood vessel, usually taken from a vein in the leg, to the surface of the heart muscle. The surgeon operates from the front of the chest; the heart is made to stop beating temporarily by using electric shock and medication. A heart-lung machine is used during this period to continue supplying blood to all parts of

175

the body. One end of the vein in the leg is attached to the aorta, the main blood vessel coming from the heart. The other end is stitched to the heart beyond the obstructed area of the old artery.

Another approach is to use the internal mammary artery, and artery supplying blood to your breast. This artery is small and delicate, and it takes longer to operate if the surgeon is performing an internal mammary artery bypass operation. Better long-term results, with much lower chances of re-stenosis, have been reported with this technique. However, if a patient urgently requires a bypass operation, the leg vein operation is more commonly performed. Due to the better long-term results, many surgeons feel that, whenever possible, an internal mammary bypass should be performed.

Dangers of Bypass Surgery: Although the technique of bypass surgery has improved over the past fifteen years, the surgery is not completely free from complications. Some of the common problems are as below:

Heart attack: Despite great attention usually given to the stitching of the grafted vein, a small area of obstruction may result in damage to the heart muscle and possibly lead to a heart attack. Since all patients are normally under close supervision after the surgery, most patients survive these heart attacks.

Confusion and disorientation: Although the blood supply to the brain is maintained without interruption, the psychological effects of surgery are not always easy to avoid. Between 5-10% of patients may experience a period of confusion and disorientation following bypass surgery. Fortunately, there is no permanent brain damage and as the patient gets better medically, normal mental functions return within a few days.

High blood pressure: Cardiac surgery is a major stress. Due to the secretion of excessive stress hormones—catecholamines and renin—from the nerves and the kidneys, the blood pressure rises temporarily in upto 30% of all bypass surgery patients. Close medical supervision is essential for controlling the blood pressure.

Irregular heart beats: Coronary heart disease itself can cause all types of irregular heartbeats. For the first few days, bypass patients are particularly at risk of irregular heartbeats. Most bypass surgery centres prefer to limit visits of family members and friends in order to avoid the risk of infection and emotional stress. Close medical supervision remains important for the control of all types of irregular heart beats.

Re-stenosis: The recurrence of narrowing and clogging of the grafted vessel, whether a vein or artery, is a major problem. It is essential to remember that bypass surgery is not the final answer to the problem of coronary heart disease. Yes, for a certain period, you have a new blood vessel that can maintain the blood supply to your heart. But the long-term solutions lie in the prevention of atherosclerosis and re-stenosis of the newly-grafted blood vessels.

Percutaneous Transluminal Coronary Angioplasty (PTCA) or Balloon Angioplasty

Percutaneous Transluminal Coronary Angioplasty (PTCA) was first developed by Dr Andreas Gruntzig in 1977, in Zurich, Switzerland. Today, well over 250,000 angioplasties are done in the United States alone each year. Like many other techniques, the PTCA success rate has improved consistently over the past ten years. PTCA is used for patients who do not respond satisfactorily to medical treatment and yet do not quite require a full-fledged bypass operation, such as someone with one or two diseased vessels, or someone whose symptoms indicate a blockage that is easily rectifiable with balloon angioplasty.

In this procedure, a catheter with an attached ballon is passed into the arteries of the heart. When the tip of the catheter reaches the area of the blockage in the coronary artery, the balloon is blown up and the plaque in the wall of the artery is pressed. Just like the bypass procedure, the symptoms of angina are likely to get better after the area of narrowing in the coronary artery has been dilated by the use of the balloon.

In the case of patients whose general health makes them unfit for a bypass operation, balloon angioplasty is a much simpler way of treatment. If a patient who has had bypass surgery several years ago, develops re-stenosis and is too ill to stand another major bypass surgery, he may also benefit from balloon angioplasty.

Despite its widespread use, PTCA has its own limitations. In some patients with a significant coronary artery blockage, the catheter or guide wire may be difficult to pass beyond the area of narrowing. In other cases, if over a prolonged period, the narrowing has developed into a hard and rigid constriction, this procedure may fail to sufficiently dilate the area of narrowing. In approximately five per cent of patients, the abrupt closure of the dilated area may require urgent bypass surgery. Since re-stenosis of coronary arteries remains a real problem, patients undergoing PTCA must change their lifestyle and ensure that their cholesterol levels are maintained within normal limits at all times.

Implantation of Stents

In 1969, Dottler and his colleagues used stainless steel coils to unblock the narrowing of the peripheral arteries of the dog. Several designs of stainless steel or tentalum stents have recently been developed and these include the spring-loaded balloon, as well as expandable and thermal memory stents. Except for their technical differences, the goal of all stents is to overcome the commonly associated problems of PTCA, that is, the failure of dilatation of coronary arteries, sudden closure and re-stenosis. In a recent study presented at the annual American Heart Association meeting in Atlanta, United States, researchers from Netherlands concluded that a reduced re-stenosis rate was the single most important advantage of using stents when compared to PTCA. Clot formation or thrombosis, and infection are the two most common complications of stent implantation. Although the overall safety of a stent operation is comparable to PTCA, this technique still remains in its early stages and, therefore, more experience and studies are required to assess the precise safety and success of this procedure.

Coronary Atherectomy

The arterial narrowing in atherectomy procedures is opened up by displacing or removing the area of the plaque. Atherectomy is particularly helpful for patients whose coronary arteries are not easily amenable to treatment with PTCA. Patients returning with re-stenosis after PTCA, or those who have ulcerated or eccentric plaques, or long and angulated areas of narrowing, are also considered to be suitable candidates for this procedure. Selected patients with a significant narrowing at the origin of coronary arteries (ostial lesions), or those suffering from complete blockage of arteries, are also likely to benefit from atherectomy.

At least four different types of procedures have been developed and these include the directional coronary atherectomy, the transluminal extraction, the flexible rotational atherectomy system and the transluminal lysing system. The plaque removal in all these systems is achieved through high-speed rotation of the device. The design and the size of the catheter, as well as the cutting head and speed of rotation vary with each procedure. The Rotablator, Simpson Atherocath and the Kensey Catheters are three of the popular systems in use. The selection of the procedure depends on the extent of narrowing of the coronary arteries. The Rotablator is particularly useful for long calcified areas of narrowing of the arteries. Unfortunately many of the complications of atherectomy are similar to those of PTCA: abrupt closure, sudden heart attack and perforation of the artery. As of now, it seems that atherectomy only has a limited use for selected patients. However, with the improvement of the technique, atherectomy may offer more than what PTCA can achieve.

Laser Angioplasty

Laser surgery is being developed for many medical problems. Although still in its early stages, the future seems to be very promising for laser surgery. In its early days it was thought that laser technology would completely eliminate the need for using guide wires to open up the blocked coronary arteries. However, it has been noted that for successful laser angioplasty, the clogged coronary arteries must first be traversed by a catheter. Laser angioplasty is being increasingly used in specialized centres for selected patients with long, diffused areas of blockage and/or eccentric and irregular plaques. Unfortunately the rate of recurrence of narrowing (re-stenosis) is not significantly different with laser angioplasty as compared to PTCA. Perforation of the coronary artery is also a known complication of laser treatment.

While balloon angioplasty has become a well-established procedure, newer techniques to unblock the coronary arteries are being developed. In approximately 3-12% of patients, mostly with severe occlusions, if the physician employs the use of PTCA, he is either unable to pass the catheter, or fails to adequately dilate the area of blockage. Newer procedures such as directional coronary atherectomy, stent implantation and laser angioplasty are expected to provide an important alternative for treatment in these patients. Nevertheless, the increasing use of balloon angioplasty will still remain the mainstay of treatment for most patients with blocked coronary arteries.

30

Prevent a Second Heart Attack

In everything the middle course is best; all things in excess bring trouble.

PLAUTUS

Fortunately the percentage of people surviving a heart attack has improved steadily. Twenty years ago, up to 50% people died within the first week of their heart attack. Now up to 70% of patients are able to survive after the first heart attack. Of the 700,000 patients with heart attacks that are admitted to the hospital each year in the United States alone, approximately 550,000 survive, and are discharged from the hospitals. Increasing awareness of the disease, better diagnosis and improved medical facilities are some of the reasons why more people are able to survive their heart attacks today as compared to twenty years ago.

Although heart attack remains a dreaded disease, you can easily find people around you who had a heart attack some five to fifteen years ago and are still leading a good quality of life. During my childhood, I had a chance to know a *Vaidji*, an Ayurvedic physician, who, I was told, had had a heart attack some twenty years earlier. He survived for at least another twenty years since I first met him. In other words, he was able to survive for at least forty more years after his heart attack. Most people who knew the *Vaidji* closely,

181

agreed that he had led a very peaceful lifestyle. He followed a simple vegetarian diet, walked 5-7 km regularly, and never lost his temper. What can we learn from this short story?

First of all, the simple fact is that you can expect to live for many years even if you have suffered a heart attack. Your lifestyle has a lot to do with your survival, especially after the heart attack. It is not as if these things are less important for those who have remained free of heart attack. Even in the absence of a heart attack, with advancing age, your coronary arteries continue to narrow as a result of slow deposition of fat and cholesterol. Therefore, it is essential to do something that would stop or even reverse the process of hardening and narrowing (atherosclerosis) of the coronary arteries.

Admittedly, your chances of getting a second heart attack are somewhat higher if you have already suffered your first heart attack. However, do not forget that someone else of your age may have a far severe degree of coronary artery disease, and may not even survive his first heart attack. The fact that you have already survived your first heart attack should make you pause and think about some of the important changes that you can bring into your life.

Ten Important Steps to Safeguard Your Health

The following are the ten most important steps that you, the survivor of the first heart attack, will find most helpful:

1. Change your attitude towards your health.

Many people who have suffered a heart attack continue to ignore the basic facts about a healthy heart. Based on scientific facts, your physician can tell you if you are at a high, medium or low risk for another heart attack. It is quite likely that in the years before your first heart attack, you failed to give due attention to reducing your risk of heart disease. Anyway, it is never too late to start! Remember, you are never too old to stop smoking, start exercising, and taking the right diet. Many heart attack survivors and their family members, unfortunately, forget that even after a heart attack, a person can live for many years. Some continue to believe wrongly that another heart attack and death is not far away. This kind of attitude is simply a sign of lack of knowledge. With a sensible lifestyle you can expect to live long enough to enjoy the company of your grandchildren. Do not consider a second heart attack and premature death as inevitable. Develop a positive attitude and tell yourself: 'Perhaps I failed to follow the rules for living a healthy life before. I will not let myself become a victim of another heart attack. With a new approach to life, I am ready to live and have fun!'

2. Stop smoking if you have not already done so.

The chances are that you were warned by your doctor at the time of your first heart attack against smoking. Smoking can increase your chances of a second heart attack substantially.

3. Make dietary changes now.

When I think of the premature heart attacks and the deaths of some of my close family members, I often think of their diets which were almost always full of fried food, excessive calories and plenty of *desi ghee*. It is no wonder that they were overweight as well. Reduce the intake of calories, saturated fat and cholesterol in your diet.

4. Reduce body weight to your normal range.

Excessive body weight poses a serious problem and increases your risk of a second heart attack.

5. Start with a regular physical exercise programme.

Scientific studies have confirmed that even after a heart attack, those who exercise regularly have a 24-32% better chance of living longer than those who do not exercise. In one study report, a moderate amount of exercise through easy, leisure-time activities such as gardening, yard work, home repairs and dancing, was associated with a 30% reduction in deaths of middle-aged men over a period of 7 years after the first heart attack. Although you can achieve a good cardiac benefit by exercising for 30-40 minutes, 3-4 times a week, I normally suggest that heart-attack patients exercise daily.

6. Reduce the stress in your life.

Excessive stress causes chemical changes that are harmful

to your heart. Stress also tends to increase your blood cholesterol. Those with a *Type B personality,* that is, with a relaxed lifestyle, have a lower risk of heart disease as compared to those with *Type A personality,* that is, those with a stressful lifestyle.

7. Give due attention to co-existing diseases.

Many heart-attack patients tend to have one or more of the problems including hypertension, diabetes mellitus and high cholesterol. Poor control of blood sugar, blood pressure and blood cholesterol can lead to a second heart attack.

8. Know your medications well.

Many heart-attack patients are discharged from the hospital and put on several different drugs. All drugs have serious side-effects. Maintain a list of proper doses, the purpose of use and the side-effects of all drugs you are taking. If you are suspecting any side-effects, discuss them with your doctor. Aspirin has been reported to decrease the risk of a second heart attack by as much as 50%. If you are not already taking aspirin for prevention of a second heart attack, go and see your doctor today.

9. Discuss the use of alcohol with your doctor.

If you have been drinking in the past, it is not safe to start drinking for the first few weeks after your heart attack. The recovery of the damaged heart muscle takes several weeks. Excessive drinking is not good for the heart but your doctor may allow you to resume moderate drinking by taking one or two drinks per day after six to eight weeks.

10. Discuss any questions regarding sex after a heart attack with your doctor.

Most heart-attack patients are able to resume their sexual activity within four to six weeks of the heart attack. For some who continue to get irregular heart beats or symptoms of heart failure, appropriate treatment with medication is essential. The fear that sexual activity may bring on a sudden heart attack has been found to be only a myth.

During the past thirty years, the outlook for recovery and survival after the first heart attack has improved significantly.

In 1958, when my uncle had a heart attack at the age of thirty-two, the best heart specialists advised complete bedrest for at least three months. Today the regimen of heart-attack patients has changed dramatically. Patients are encouraged to walk as early as the second or third day after the heart attack. Most patients are discharged after seven to ten days from the hospital. Our thinking and attitudes have undergone radical changes. Now heart-attack patients are normally asked to return to their work within a few weeks. Most heart attack patients continue to lead a normal life for decades after their heart attack.

Even if you have already suffered a heart attack, there is every reason for you to think in terms of living a long life. This can, however, be achieved only if you are willing to make necessary changes in your diet and lifestyle.

Post-operative Care

Hundreds of bypass operations are carried out each month in India alone. However, bypass surgery is not the final answer. About forty-five per cent of bypass grafts can close up in one year, forty to fifty per cent in five years, and seventy per cent of the severely damaged arteries in seven years. Therefore, steps to change the lifestyle are more important in patients who have already undergone bypass surgery

If, for example, a patient continues to smoke after surgery, the newly-grafted vessel may even be occluded within 3-5 years, thus making another surgical operation necessary. Many surgeons are not even enthusiastic about operating on someone who is not willing to stop smoking. Dietary changes are of the utmost importance. Several studies have confirmed that a low cholesterol and low fat diet is helpful for the prevention of re-stenosis, that is narrowing and clogging of the grafted blood vessels.

Aggressive lowering of cholesterol can make a significant difference in the long-term success of a bypass heart operation. A major study, the Cholesterol Lowering Atherosclerosis Study (CLAS) involved 162 men who had previously undergone coronary artery bypass surgery. As a result of aggressive treatment with diet and cholesterol-lowering drugs (niacin and cholestyramine), cholesterol reduction of 25%, LDL reduction of 43%, and HDL rise of 37% was noted. More than 16% of patients showed a reversal of atherosclerosis on angiography; only 3.6% patients treated with diet alone showed some improvement in atherosclerosis on angiography. In total, 61% patients treated with diet and cholesterol-lowering drugs remained stable or improved significantly as compared to only 40% on diet treatment alone. The conclusion was that cholesterol reduction is very helpful for preventing the re-stenosis.

Intensive cholesterol lowering has also been noted to delay the recurrence of stenosis after percutaneous transluminal coronary angioplasty (PTA). Study results presented at the annual meeting of the American College of Cardiologists by Dr Zua-Qiao Zhao, of the University of Washington, confirms the role of cholesterol-lowering in PTCA patients. Six months after successful PTCA, 16 patients were divided into 3 subgroups. Group A received cholesterol-lowering medication—niacin and cholestyramine; group B also received cholesterol-lowering medication—cholestyramine and lovastatin; and the third group did not receive any medication. After a period of two and a half years, Dr Zhao noted that the re-stenosis was much less in those receiving treatment for reduction of cholesterol, that is, groups A and B. In the group that had high cholesterol values, there was a worsening of symptoms, and many of these patients required a repeat PTCA procedure.

The same steps that are important for someone who has already had a heart attack, are also important for patients who have already undergone bypass surgery. Cessation of smoking, regular exercise, reduction of stress, and a low fat and low cholesterol diet are some of the important steps for patients who have already undergone PTCA or bypass surgery. Although surgical techniques do improve the quality of life for heart disease patients, they cannot be considered a complete cure for the problem of coronary heart disease.

31

The Future is Alive & Healthy

My interest is in the future because I am going to spend the rest of my life there.

CHARLES F. KETTERING

Although coronary heart disease still remains a major killer, we have been able to clearly identify its risk factors. Several risk factors like heredity, high blood pressure, smoking, diabetes and obesity have been known for a long time. Although high cholesterol has been suspected to be a culprit for a number of years, it is mainly during the past ten years that we have come to recognize cholesterol as a major risk factor for coronary heart disease.

Unlike genetic risks that you simply cannot change, reducing cholesterol is all within your own control. Research has confirmed, beyond any doubt, that high blood cholesterol level increases your risk of coronary heart disease. Not only that, it has been shown that with each 1% reduction of cholesterol level, you can cut down your risk of heart disease by 2%. Moreover, if you can maintain your cholesterol within lower normal limits of 150-180 mg, you can even expect to reverse the hardening of your arteries.

The dramatic reduction in the rate of death due to heart disease in the United States has been achieved mainly due to an increasing awareness on the part of the American public.

For someone who is visiting the West from India, it would not take long to see that the American people consider heart disease as their worst enemy. Compared to any other nation in the world, people in the United States are more involved in physical exercise and fitness. There are more health clubs in the United States than in any other country. People make it their business to go jogging, swimming and walking, and participating in numerous other sports activities. Millions are trying to reduce their stress through yoga and meditation. Major corporations and companies are spending millions in an effort to keep their employees healthy. Health-promoting agencies are spending a lot of money in an effort to make the people more aware of the problem of high cholesterol. As a result, the death rate due to heart disease has gone down by 40% during the past 30 years.

Unfortunately, many people in India remain ignorant about the principles of good health until they themselves are affected by heart disease. Most people continue to believe that they will somehow escape from the disease and if anything bad is to happen, it will happen to somebody else. As a result of this unfortunate thinking, many keep postponing taking any serious steps for good health. If you really want to enjoy many years of healthy living, good health has to be your high priority. Good health does not happen automatically! Like many other things in life, you have to plan and work hard to achieve fitness.

All of us learned many years ago that ignorance of the law is no excuse. Ignorance or awareness, particularly in the area of health maintenance, can make or break your life. We have to understand a simple concept. Most scientists now firmly believe that nature has designed the human body to last for, at least, 110-120 years. It is only this type of thinking that has led people in the West to look very seriously at the leading causes of death, and take steps to prevent premature deaths due to common causes such as heart disease. What has been achieved as a result of these efforts is worth looking into. At the beginning of this century, an average child born in the West could expect to live only for 45 years. The same child born today can expect to live for approximately 75 years. What a wonderful achievement! Make a comparison with our own country, India. Currently, our average life expectancy is about 60 years. We are clearly at a disadvantage since an average person in the West lives for an extra 10-15 years.

Ancient Indian medicine strongly believed that the right food and a peaceful lifestyle had a lot to do with health. Dr Dean Ornish, a well-known cardiologist of San Francisco, expressed the same thoughts: 'I don't understand why asking people to eat a well-balanced vegetarian diet is considered drastic, while it is medically conservative to cut people open.' Bypass only bypasses the problem, according to him. The Ornish Plan has four major disciplines: patients adhere to a very low fat vegetarian diet, which excludes animal products except egg whites and non-fat dairy products; patients have to quit smoking; they have to practice stress management which includes yoga, meditation, positive imagery and breathing exercises, and combat emotional upheavals; they need to take up only a very moderate but regular exercise programme, which can easily be part of the daily regimen.

Ornish has been greatly influenced by the philosophy of Swami Satchidananda, ever since he came under the latter's influence in 1972. Ornish is convinced that heart disease has as much to do with one's attitudes to life, success, perceptions, ambitions, goals and one's emotional baggage.

The stress on yoga and meditation is not new to the Indian lifestyle. What is more relevant is his advocacy of a vegetarian diet that can be as varied, nutritious and adequate as it can be a potent tool to combat CHD. It is the same kind of diet that has been integral to our lifestyles for centuries but which is being widely exchanged for 'fast', fat-filled, high calorie, low nutrition foods. Ornish is convinced that cereals, legumes, vegetables and fresh fruits are far superior to fat-ridden red meats.

The first step has to be the appropriate understanding of

risk factors of CHD. Talk to your doctor today and arrange to have your cholesterol level checked. If it is found to be over 200 mg, discuss the necessary changes required in your diet and lifestyle with your physician. Remember, high blood cholesterol does not necessarily mean taking tablets for the rest of your life. Fortunately, in most cases, sensible changes in the diet, concentration on low fat and low cholesterol, putting an end to smoking, a regular exercise programme, and lowering your body weight and stress level are all that you require to lower your risk of heart attack. But do not delay this any longer. Any ignorance or neglect on your part may prove to be life-threatening.

Many people have succeeded in making these simple changes. After an initial discomfort, you may, indeed, find that you are enjoying your rejuvenated lifestyle. The new strength and stamina that will flow through your arteries, muscles and bones will, undoubtedly, help your cardiovascular system and save you from the disaster of a heart attack. Many people, unfortunately, wait for a heart attack to occur before they are convinced that they should change their lifestyle. It has been said that, whereas, a person with an average intelligence learns from his own mistakes, a wise person always learns from the mistakes of others. However, a foolish person fails to learn from either. Do what the wise people do. The importance of knowing and reducing your cholesterol cannot be over-emphasized. The penalty of ignorance is sudden death due to a heart attack—a penalty that is just too high to ignore!

32

Common Questions about Cholesterol

Doctors are always working to preserve our health and cooks to destroy it, but the latter are often more successful.

DENIS DIDEROT

It is not only people living in cosmopolitan cities like Delhi, Bombay or Calcutta who are affected by heart attacks; even those living in small towns and villages are becoming increasingly prone to them.

Commonly asked questions regarding cholesterol and its relationship with heart attacks are discussed below:

Q. *I have heard of cholesterol. Is any amount safe?*

A. Adults must not have more than 200 mg of cholesterol per 100 ml of blood. Unfortunately, between 30-50% of all American adults have higher levels of cholesterol that increase their risk of heart attacks.

Q. *I am confused about the benefit of monounsaturated versus polyunsaturated fat. Which one is better? Please explain.*

A. All unsaturated fats, including monounsaturated and polyunsaturated are better than saturated fats. Rich sources of polyunsaturated fat are corn, soya bean, safflower and sunflower oil. Monounsaturated fat is found in high amounts in olive, canola and peanut oil. It is believed that monounsaturated fat provides more protection to your heart as compared to polyunsaturated fat.

Q. *I am 25 years old and my cholesterol level is 192 mg. I like a two-egg omlette every day. Since my cholesterol is normal, is it safe to continue eating an omlette daily?*

A. Although your cholesterol, being below 200 mg, is within normal limits, your daily cholesterol consumption is between 500-600 mg. Each egg contains between 250-300 mg of cholesterol. It is recommended that one should limit the cholesterol intake to less than 300 mg per day. It has been established that with advancing years of life our cholesterol tends to rise. If you do not cut down your cholesterol intake now, there are high chances that your cholesterol level will be more than 200 mg within the next few years. A low cholesterol and low fat diet is advisable for all including those who have normal cholesterol levels. A good approach will be to limit your intake of eggs to 4-6 eggs per week. One more suggestion is to discard the yellow part of the egg if you still wish to consume two or more eggs per day. It is the central, yellow part of the egg that contains all cholesterol. The egg white contains all the protein.

Q. *My father had a heart attack that killed him at the age of 46. Am I also at an increased risk of having a heart attack?*

A. Many common diseases including diabetes, heart attack, asthma and arthritis have a genetic predisposition, that is, there is a tendency for these conditions to be passed on to their children. If one or both parents happen to suffer from the disease, the risk is greater for the children. Of course, if both parents were affected, the chances are higher as compared to only one parent being affected. Remember, with a positive family history, even though your chances are somewhat increased, there is no need to panic! There is a lot that you can do to minimize your risk of heart attack. Hereditary or genetic components are just one of the many risk factors. Simple lifestyle changes can substantially reduce your chances of having a heart attack.

Q. *What is 'good' and 'bad' cholesterol?*

A. Total cholesterol, if over 200 mg, is considered to be harmful and increases your risk of heart attack. There are two main types of cholesterol: high density lipoprotein (HDL), also referred to as 'good' cholesterol; and low density lipoprotein (LDL), also known as 'bad' cholesterol. The normal level of HDL is 40-65 mg. HDL protects the heart against heart attacks. Women tend to have higher levels of HDL than men. In general, the higher the concentration of HDL, the better it is for your heart. LDL levels must not exceed 130 mg. The higher the LDL, the worse it is for your heart. Another type of cholesterol is called triglyceride. The normal level for triglycerides is between 100-200 mg. High levels of triglycerides are also damaging to the heart.

Q. *What can I do to raise my levels of HDL?*

A. HDL is a good form of cholesterol that can protect you from heart disease. As such, there is no single 'best' step that you can take to increase your HDL. However, higher levels of HDL are commonly found in people who do not smoke, exercise regularly and maintain normal body weight.

Q. *Can high levels of triglycerides also cause heart disease?*

A. Triglyceride is a form of fat that has recently been recognized to increase your risk of heart disease. In a normal adult, the total fasting triglyceride must not exceed 200 mg. People with high triglyceride level are often found to have high total and LDL cholesterol, and lower HDL cholesterol. Steps that would normally lower the total cholesterol are usually effective in lowering the triglyceride level.

Q. *What is the effect of lifestyle on blood cholesterol level?*

A. Your lifestyle and dietary habits have a lot to do with your cholesterol level. The following elements of your lifestyle can cause high cholesterol: smoking, lazy lifestyle, high fat and high cholesterol diet, high stress level and excessive alcohol intake.

Q. *Doctors often talk about regular exercise being good for your heart. Can regular exercise lower my cholesterol as well?*

A. If you are physically active, your chances of getting a heart attack are much lower. Regular exercise can reduce your cholesterol and even increase your HDL or good cholesterol. Physical exercise leads to improved blood supply to the heart. Those who exercise regularly have wide coronary arteries. Exercise also helps in keeping the blood pressure within normal range. Further, exercise also helps in losing excessive body weight which, indirectly, improves the efficiency of the heart. Even those who have already suffered a heart attack can expect to live longer and even avoid a second heart attack by following a programme of regular exercise. However, before you start exercising vigorously, check with your doctor. Strenuous exercise may not be the best thing for you if you are not accustomed to exercising. Particularly for those who are over the age of thirty-five years, a SLOW START with a gradual increase in the amount of exercise is advised.

Q. *I have been taking good care of my diet; yet, my cholesterol remains around 235 mg. Does it mean that I am still at risk of having a heart attack?*

A. Unfortunately, the answer is 'yes'. Your efforts in reducing your fat and cholesterol intake may be worth applauding. Yet it seems it is not working enough to bring your cholesterol down to 200 mg. The fact is that you must not allow the cholesterol to go above a 200 mg level. First, discuss your diet with your doctor and see if he can suggest some more changes that might help you to reduce your cholesterol level further. The dietary changes must be tried for at least six months before starting any medication to lower the cholesterol. Fortunately, if the dietary efforts fail to achieve the desirable level of cholesterol, there are currently a number of drugs available; one or more of these can help you to successfully lower your cholesterol.

33

Test Your Understanding

If a man empties his purse into his head, no man can take it away from him. An investment in knowledge always pays the best interest.

BENJAMIN FRANKLIN

This chapter gives you an opportunity to test your own knowledge about cholesterol. Once you have answered all the questions on a separate piece of paper, check for the right answers at the end of the chapter.

For questions 1-5 put a (✓) mark against the most appropriate answer.

1. You are most likely to get a heart attack if your cholesterol is between

        a. 150-200 mg   ☐
        b. 201-239 mg   ☐
        c. 240-260 mg   ☐

2. You are more likely to get a heart attack if your HDL cholesterol is between

        a. 25-29 mg   ☐
        b. 30-35 mg   ☐
        c. 36-45 mg   ☐

3. Your risk of heart attack is highest if your LDL cholesterol is between

              a. 100-129 mg   ☐
              b. 130-159 mg   ☐
              c. 160-190 mg   ☐

4. You are more likely to get a heart attack if your triglyceride level is

              a. < 200 mg   ☐
              b. 200-400 mg   ☐
              c. 401-600 mg   ☐

5. Regular intake of *Isapgol* can

              a. lower your cholesterol   ☐
              b. raise your blood sugar   ☐
              c. cause stomach ulcers   ☐

6. One egg contains approximately 300 mg of cholesterol.

              True   ☐
              False   ☐

7. If you have diabetes mellitus, you are more likely to have a high cholesterol level.

              True   ☐
              False   ☐

8. If you are already taking drugs to lower the cholesterol, you do not need to worry about your diet control.

              True   ☐
              False   ☐

9. A stressful lifestyle can increase your blood cholesterol.

              True   ☐
              False   ☐

10. High intake of carrots can reduce your risk of coronary heart disease.

              True   ☐
              False   ☐

11. High blood cholesterol, smoking and high blood pressure are the three most important risk factors for heart disease.

              True   ☐
              False   ☐

12. If you stop taking any cholesterol in your diet, you will not have any cholesterol in your blood.

True	☐
False	☐

13. Doing regular physical exercise can reduce your blood cholesterol.

True	☐
False	☐

14. Butter and *desi ghee* are rich sources of saturated fat.

True	☐
False	☐

15. High cholesterol is dangerous only for adults; children and older people do not need to worry about taking high cholesterol diets.

True	☐
False	☐

16. By lowering your blood cholesterol you can even reverse the process of narrowing and hardening of coronary arteries.

True	☐
False	☐

17. Eating fish at least twice a week can reduce your risk of heart attack.

True	☐
False	☐

18. Having bypass heart surgery gives you permanent protection from heart disease.

True	☐
False	☐

19. Thin people do not really need to have their blood cholesterol checked because they hardly have any risk of heart disease.

True	☐
False	☐

20. Drinking beer is better than taking whisky or hard drinks for your heart.

True	☐
False	☐

Now, check and see if your answers are correct or not.

Answers:

1=c.

Many studies have confirmed a close relationship of high cholesterol with an increased incidence of coronary heart disease. If your cholesterol is over 200 mg, you have an increased risk of heart disease. People with a cholesterol level of over 240 mg are particularly at a greater risk.

2=a.

HDL, the 'good' cholesterol, helps to transport the cholesterol back to your liver and then out of your body through the digestive system. People with high HDL levels enjoy greater protection from coronary heart disease. If your HDL level is below 30 mg, you are especially at a greater risk of developing heart disease.

3=c.

LDL, the 'bad' cholesterol, increases your risk of heart disease. The higher the LDL level, the greater is your risk. A normal LDL level means that your LDL should not be over 130 mg.

4=c.

In a normal adult, the triglyceride levels must not be over 200 mg. Triglycerides are one of the types of fat in your blood. The word 'tri' stands for 3 fatty acid chains. These chains are attached with glycerol in triglyceride and, hence, the term triglyceride. Research has now proved that if you have high triglyceride in your blood, you are at a greater risk of heart disease.

5=a.

Isapgol is a rich source of fibre. Regular use of *Isapgol* (1-2 tablespoonfuls) can not only help you prevent constipation, but also lower your blood cholesterol by 10-20%. I strongly suggest that you take *Isapgol* regularly even if you have no problem with your bowel habits.

6=True.

One large egg contains between 250-300 mg of cholesterol. It is recommended that you should limit your daily cholesterol intake to less than 300 mg per day.

7=True.

More than 50% of diabetic patients have high cholesterol levels. If your diabetes is poorly controlled, your chances of having high cholesterol are very high. Since both high blood sugar and blood cholesterol can increase your risk of heart disease, it is essential that you seek the help of your physician for better control of diabetes as well as high cholesterol.

8=False.

A reduced intake of fat and cholesterol in your diet remains the most important part of treatment for anyone with high cholesterol levels. For most patients who can significantly lower their fat and cholesterol intake, there is no need to take any cholesterol-lowering medication.

9 = True.

Stressful lifestyle, through various chemical changes in your body, can increase your cholesterol level.

10=True.

Research has shown that foods containing beta-carotene and vitamins C and E can protect your heart from coronary artery disease. Carrots are a rich source of beta-carotene.

11=True.

Although there are many risk factors (genetics, obesity, physical inactivity and diabetes mellitus), high blood cholesterol, high blood pressure and smoking are the three most important risk factors for coronary heart disease.

12=False.

Besides dietary cholesterol intake, cholesterol is constantly produced by your liver. Your body cells require small amounts of cholesterol for proper functioning. Even if you completely stop taking cholesterol in your diet, your liver can successfully manage to meet your body's cholesterol needs at all times.

13=True.

Physical exercise has many benefits including reduction of body weight, blood cholesterol and blood pressure. Exercise also leads to dilatation of the coronary arteries. Those who exercise regularly have much lower chances of heart attacks.

14=True.

Butter and *desi ghee* are rich sources of saturated fat. You can definitely reduce your risk of heart disease by reducing your intake of saturated fat.

15=False.

High cholesterol can cause significant damage to coronary arteries in people of all ages. In fact, the process of coronary heart disease or atherosclerosis starts early in childhood. It is only through lifelong preventive steps that you can expect to remain free of heart disease.

16=True.

Studies have shown that by changing your diet and lifestyle, you can reverse the damage that has already been done to your coronary arteries. A low fat and low cholesterol diet, regular exercise and reduction of stress can help you reverse the process of coronary heart disease.

17=True.

Recent scientific studies have confirmed that those who consume fish at least twice a week are less prone to get heart attacks.

18=False.

By having a new blood vessel grafted in your heart, you can expect to be free of chest pain and shortness of breath for a few years. Unfortunately, bypass surgery does not provide you with a permanent solution. If you fail to take the right steps, the new blood vessel in your heart can become clogged once again.

19=False.

Heart disease has many risk factors and being overweight is just one of them. In general, thin people tend to have normal cholesterol levels and are, thus, at a lower risk of heart disease. Yet, a thin person who has a stressful lifestyle and is a smoker remains at a high risk of developing heart disease.

20=False.

Excessive alcohol intake in any form, including beer, whisky, wine, vodka and rum is bad for your heart, liver, brain, and the nerves. However, it has been noted that moderate drinkers, that is, those who take one to two drinks per day, are at a lower risk of developing coronary heart disease.

Glossary

Anabolic Steroids: Any of a group of steroid hormones produced by the adrenal glands and used to increase muscle strength.

Androgenic Hormones: Substances capable of developing and maintaining certain male sexual characteristics.

Angina: Chest pain or discomfort on physical exertion. Typically the pain disappears on taking rest or a glyceryl trinitrate tablet.

Angioplasty: Percutaneous transluminal coronary angioplasty (PTCA) is often referred to as angioplasty or ballooning. A catheter tube is introduced into the narrowed coronary artery where it is ballooned up to widen the narrowed coronary artery.

Arrhythmia: Arrhythmia is said to exist if the heartbeat is not regular. Irregular heartbeats may result from irregular contractions of upper or lower chambers, the atria or the ventricles.

Arterioles: Smaller arteries.

Atherosclerosis: The narrowing and hardening of arteries due to cholesterol and fat deposition on the wall of the arteries.

Beta-blockers: Drugs that prevent the stimulation of increased cardiac action. They are used to treat angina and reduce high blood pressure.

Beta-carotene: It is a naturally occuring pigment in plant products such as spinach, carrots, oranges, etc. Beta-carotene protects the cells from becoming cancerous.

Bypass Operation: A common surgical procedure used for coronary heart disease patients. A new pipe, a vein, is attached to the heart to bypass the area of the blocked coronary artery.

Catheter: A tube for insertion into a body cavity for introducing or removing fluid.

Cellulose: A carbohydrate forming the main constitutent of plant cell-walls.

Cholesterol: A hard waxy substance that is found in foods of animals origin. Within the body the liver also produces cholesterol.

Coronary Angiography: A special X-ray technique in which a dye is injected into the coronary arteries to diagnose the exact location and extent of the narrowing of arteries.

Coronary Arteries: The arteries that supply the heart muscle with oxygen.

Coronary Artery Disease: Also known as Coronary heart disease and ischaemic heart disease. The narrowing of the coronary arteries results in reduced blood supply to the heart muscle, impairing its functioning. The symptoms include chest pain, shortness of breath, and tiredness on moderate exertion.

Cortico Steroids: A kind of organic compound produced in the cortex of the adrenal gland.

Delirium Tremens: Hallucinations and tremors produced in the body, generally due to chronic alchoholism.

Diabetes Mellitus: A common disease in which the patient has high blood sugar. Since sugar is wasted in urine and the body cells cannot utilize sugar properly, the patients feel weak and tired, and have higher chances of infections and other complications.

Diastole: The period of heart relaxation. The heart contracts at regular intervals. Contraction is referred to as systole.

Diuretics: Drugs that lead to excessive loss of water and electrolytes (sodium, chloride and potassium) from the body. Diuretics decrease the water load, and are therefore commonly used for hypertension and heart failure:

Electrocardiography (ECG): The small amount of electric current generated by the heart is recorded by the ECG tracing which enables diagnosis of several conditions of the heart.

Estrogen: A hormone developing and maintaining female characteristics of the body.

Exercise Stress Test: An ECG-type of recording system monitors how well your heart can cope with the extra work load when exercising. Thallium, a radio-opaque material, may also be used in some cases.

Heart Attack: Myocardial infarction is the medical term for heart attack. A part of the heart muscle is damaged because of the complete blockage of the coronary artery.

Heart Failure: Heart failure is said to exist if your heart cannot beat strong enough to maintain sufficient blood supply to all parts of your body.

Holter Monitor: A sophisticated test that records your heartbeat for a prolonged period (24-48 hours) and can help your doctor to find out whether your heart beats regularly at all times or not, including when you are walking, working or sleeping.

Hypertension: The blood pressure is expressed in 2 numbers, the systolic and the diastolic. The systolic is the upper number (when your heart is contracting); the diastolic is the lower number (when your heart is relaxing). The normal adult reading is systolic 110-140 mm, and diastolic 60-90 mm. If your systolic blood pressure is over 150 mm, and/or diastolic is over 90 mm, you probably suffer from hypertension, i.e. high blood pressure.

Lignin: A complex organic compound deposited in the cell-walls of many plants.

Lipids: Lipids are types of fat that get deposited in the walls of the arteries and cause narrowing and hardening of the arteries.

Mucilage: A sticky, semi-fluid substance obtained from plant seeds, etc, by soaking them.

Myocardial Infarction: *See Heart Attack*

Myocardial Ischaemia: Reduced blood supply to the heart muscle.

Myocardium: This is the main muscular layer of the heart. The inner lining of the heart is called endocardium and the outer sac is called the pericardium.

Oat Bran: The husk separated from the oat plant.

Pectins: Soluble gelatinous carbohydrate compounds found in ripe fruits, etc.

Plaque: Small plates of fat and cholesterol that are deposited in the walls of the arteries.

Platelets: The blood has 3 main types of cells. The red blood cells (RBCs) carry oxygen, white blood cells (WBCs) fight infections, and platelets—cells that come into action for plugging and forming a blood clot.

Pulmonary Embolism: An obstruction of any blood vessel due to a blood clot or air bubble in the lungs.

Re-stenosis: The recurrent narrowing of a passage in the body.

Silent Heart Disease: This is said to exist if a person has no significant chest pain, yet the heart muscle does not receive sufficient blood supply. It may kill without any warning.

Systole: The contraction of the heart muscle.

Thrombosis: Coagulation of blood in a vein or artery.

Triglycerides: A form of fat.

Vasodilators: Medicines which cause dilatation of the blood vessels.

Index